SO YOU WANT TO BE THIN

Then Use
F.A.T.

by
Billy Branson

ISBN-13: 978-1495439841

ISBN-10: 1495439844

Version 2.14.14X2

Also available in eBook

Cover design by

Gordon A Kessler
and Vicki Ellis

Disclaimer: This book is intended for educational purposes only and not to be construed as medical advice or diagnosis. The author assumes no responsibility for misuse of the materials provided herein. Consult your doctor before changing dietary intake or beginning a new exercise program. Even walking can be dangerous if you are extremely overweight.

The author cannot be responsible for broken or disconnected Internet links.

Dedicated to all the overweight people of this world.

SPECIAL THANKS TO:

Venice Hunter
Vicki Ellis
Gordon Kessler

iv

TABLE OF CONTENTS

FOREWORD

Weight control has become almost a daily topic of conversation everywhere. Why? Because a lot of people have come to the realization that excess fat is neither healthy nor becoming to them.

In my case, excess weight would prevent my being able to walk; I am one of the physically challenged. My personal concern with weight began soon after an auto accident back in 1950. That accident paralyzed me. I awakened my body over the years but walking is still difficult. The less weight I have to carry around, the easier it is to walk.

And there are a growing number of physically challenged and elderly people in this world who, like me, can't run, jog, or even walk fast. We can't exercise enough to control weight. Our weight must be controlled by what we eat or don't eat. But how do we control *that*? Well, some might stay on a diet, eat certain foods, take pills, or join a how-to-lose-weight organization. But I, for one, don't intend to do that for an entire lifetime. I want to enjoy life, and one of the enjoyments of life is eating.

While wanting to enjoy ourselves, we watch TV and see the ads for foods. We watch others eat, and we shop in grocery stores. All of that may increase our food and drink desire, decrease our will power, and cause our mouths to water for much more than any of us should consume.

But despite all that, over the years I have learned how to keep my weight within ten pounds of where it should be. In fact, I usually allow only a five pound variation, up or down. And it's easy when one uses my method of weight control—the F.A.T. method found in this book.

Through many years of working with my body in order to wake it up and teach it to walk, I learned how to reprogram my mind for whatever needed to be done. In my counseling practice, I helped others make necessary changes using hypnotherapy.

During those years, I became aware of how easily my own program can be changed. Three overweight women came to see me during the same period of time, and all three wanted to weigh 125 pounds. Not remembering how relaxed and receptive I become while working with others, I hypnotized each of them on a different day of the week and had them repeat after me, "I eat the proper number of calories each day for a 125 pound woman" as one of their postulates.

Well, it wasn't long until I, too, weighed 125 pounds! And I stayed at that weight until it came to my attention that I had reprogrammed myself at the same time that I had reprogrammed the three women. So I immediately changed my thinking and dropped back down to my usual 116 pounds a couple of months later. You can believe I watched how I worded my sentences when working with others, after that!

It's not difficult to become, or maintain, the proper weight—not after you learn how. And that's why I wrote this book—so you, too, will have the know-how to be thin.

"For as he thinketh in his heart, so is he."
Proverbs 23:7

PART ONE

Patterns of Thought

Chapter One

Internal and External Agreement

Arnold is overweight—80 pounds, at least—and he has fallen in love with petite, 5'3", 110 pound Mary. All of Mary's close friends have been rather on the lean side, so Arnold feels certain she must prefer thin people like herself. At least he hasn't seen anyone, other than himself, hanging around her who is overweight. She has never been seen on a date with a fat guy.

So now Arnold tells his friends, "I want to be thin, so I'm going to lose this weight!" and then he proceeds to break a most important rule: Rule #1.

"What rule?" you ask. "I didn't know there was a set of numbered rules."

Well, maybe they're not numbered, but certainly, some are more important than others. First of all, what you say and what you think need to agree. Arnold *said* he wanted to be thin, but then he told himself, "Mary won't love me unless I'm thin, so I've got to lose weight. But I've always been fat, so it's going to be hard."

So, now we know the truth! Arnold is *really* saying, "*Mary* wants me to be thin," and, "I'm not lovable unless I'm thin."

We all do that—say one thing and think another—right? Well, maybe not *all*—there might be some perfect (?) people who always say exactly what they think. But I can remember the day

I was taught that a polite society considers such honesty rude. I was in the eighth grade of parochial school, and Sister was attempting to explain to several of us girls that, rather than offend someone, we should tell a little white lie, saying, for example, "Your dress is lovely," even when we thought it was ugly. And, if Mother wanted us to tell a would-be guest at the door that she was "not in," we could finish the sentence in our thoughts with "… to you," or we could say the opposite, "But, she really *is* in," to ourselves. That would make it okay because it was really no one's business except hers whether she was "in" or "out."

We were assured such a manipulation of our language was "*the* thing to do" in a so-called "polite society." With this new-to-me method of evasive tactics, I quickly forgot my mother's earlier teaching: "If you can't say something good, then don't say anything at all." I began to practice how many different ways I could use this *saying-one-thing-while-thinking-another*. And here I had always figured that sort of thing would be a "sin," but Sister had said it was only a "white lie" and therefore not serious.

Wow! I'd just been handed a license to *double-think-talk*!

But perhaps I grew up in a rather sheltered environment. I've since discovered most people learn much earlier than I did how this "polite" way of communicating works, and they use it often … even when "being polite" is not the objective.

Actually, you learned double-think-talk to conceal your true meanings from those with whom you converse, but you need to be aware that you may also be perplexing yourself. When the lack of internal (thinking) and external (talking) agreement has to do with your self-image, then you'd best learn to change one or the other so they agree.

Your communication is the concern of your conscious mind—the reasoning part of you. What is said or thought sinks into the subconscious mind. Think of your subconscious mind as the little "you" inside yourself, listening to everything you say, and at the same time, trying to keep track of what you're thinking. Do you have "you" confused?

You say, "What difference does it make what I say? I know I don't mean it." But the subconscious doesn't reason—that's not its job. Reasoning is the function of the conscious mind. The subconscious doesn't judge whether you mean what you say or not; it just creates from the ingredients—the patterns—you send it. The closest analogy I can think of is a computer. It works with the material you feed into it, according to a set of rules, but it doesn't decide whether this or that program is to your advantage, is correct, or is true. What comes out depends upon what goes in.

If you say to a well-meaning friend, "You're so sweet to bring me these delicious cookies," and inwardly say, "I wish she'd quit; I can't stay on a diet with all this food around!" are you hoping to deceive only her, or are you also deceiving yourself? Do you know which is the real you? Are you encouraging her to bring more food with your flattery and trying to pacify your conscience with the internal, "I wish she'd quit," or are you *really* wanting to quit eating pastries but don't want to hurt her feelings?

Are you sure?

Either way, you're going to stay fat because of your lack of internal and external agreement. You need to pay attention and become aware of your own particular pattern of double-think-talk.

If you decide to make a dress, and you say, "I want it to have long sleeves," but you think, "Short sleeves might be better; they're more comfortable," you probably won't even start cutting the material until you first decide which way you want it.

Neither will you stick to a diet or really get serious about losing that weight until you come to an agreement with yourself about what your true motives are.

When there isn't an agreement, which one is likely to win

out eventually ... what you say, or what you think? Obviously, one or the other must win out. Things do change over time. But do you exert any conscious control over the situation? Well, probably the more emotional of the two will dominate the scene; and since thoughts create emotions—and sometimes words of one kind or another—the inner language (thoughts) wins the war of words.

For example: My mother had a rule that the older child was not allowed to hit one younger. So, no matter whether or not my younger sister hit me first, if I retaliated in kind, Mother would say (besides whatever punishment she deemed proper), "Say you're sorry." Dutifully, I would do so ... but to myself I would say, "You can make me say it, but you can't make me mean it!"

So you see, when inner and outer language do battle, it's usually the inner that wins—I definitely was not sorry! And the angry feelings persisted. Soon Old Man Resentment followed the fray by way of my being forced into the conflict in the first place.

Then too, stop and think about how we use words. We learn through association. When you were small, you were taught "hungry" means the stomach needs food. Now you might say, "I'm hungry for love." Earlier, you learned to associate the word "hungry" with certain internal feelings—that little gnawing, insistent, persistent ache in the pit of the stomach that screamed, "Feed me!"—and now the word, and therefore the feeling, is associated with love. Will you eat ... when it's actually love you want?

Do you *really* mean what you say? Listen to yourself. Your subconscious mind is, and it is gradually working to create what you say you want. Oh it may take a while, but nevertheless, the words have been typed in; the process has been set into motion; your computer-like subconscious mind is on automatic; and eventually, a new you will be created by way of the patterns you use.

Does your internal and external language agree? If so, then congratulations! But, if you're fat, then there is a reason you are overeating. Read on. We have only just begun to analyze Arnold ... and lots of other people who have a problem with being overweight.

Chapter Two

You Can Create a New Reality

If Arnold truly wants to be thin, he will need to become aware of another important rule, that is: You create your own reality by what you tell yourself—your own internal talkathon. Yes, we talk to ourselves all the time; it's called thinking. If we didn't, we would fall asleep or go into an altered state of consciousness— like being semi-asleep, or in a trance. So you keep on talking to yourself, and it keeps you busy creating your life ... and your size.

Your world and yourself have been described to you ever since your birth. "You're just like Uncle George!" but, you *like* your Uncle George, and Uncle George is fat. So, the message is: "Get fat and you will be just like Uncle George."

"You eat like a pig!" Your dad may have had sloppy eating habits in mind, but you may have thought, "Little piggies are *so* cute." Hadn't Porky Pig been one of your favorite cartoon animals? You could easily see him acting out a favorite scene. So you had a completely different inner vision of pigs than Dad held. And, besides, aren't pigs supposed to eat a lot and get fat? Aren't they worth more when they weigh more? But later, after you're already fat from eating everything you could get your hands on—so you'll be worth more, too—you hear pork is not good for you. Pork has too much cholesterol. And by now you've visited a farm and seen barnyard pigs that don't by any stretch of the imagination resemble old "Porky."

So now you see pigs as not-so-clean animals ... and not nearly as cute as they were when you were five years old. Then too, you've also heard, "No one loves a fatty." So you don't like yourself very much because you're fat.

But, back to Arnold, he said, "I've always been fat." Of course he's always been fat! He's been told that all his life, and he continues to tell himself that he is. In fact, he was encouraged to become fat. "Arnold will eat anything, ha-ha! Chances are he'll eat *everything* if you don't watch out! Look how much he can hold. He ate a whole pie yesterday, and I'll bet he could eat that whole cake if you let him have it!"

Yes, he got lots of attention because of his eating habits. And he needed all the attention he could get because he didn't feel very good about himself. At least, if he got attention—any kind of attention—he must be worth something! Some of his classmates got attention for showing off physically, but he wasn't at all athletic. Eating was what he'd learned to do best.

"Arnold is a good boy; he always cleans his plate," said Mother. And he wanted so much to be a "good boy," so Mother would love him. He polished his plate no matter how much was heaped upon it.

"Arnold is so fat, he split his pants when he leaned over to tie his shoe yesterday," laughed a classmate. "He was so funny; you should have seen him, ha-ha!"

Oh yes! Arnold gets lots of attention by being fat. Some of it he likes, and some of it he doesn't like—it's embarrassing; but any kind of attention is better than none.

How many homemakers receive the main compliment—attention—of their lives by way of their culinary creations? Is the extra love used to create such works of delicious art the only way some people know how to give and receive love and attention?

And think of the ways we describe little impressionable people. Seeing a roly-poly baby, someone is apt to comment, "She's so cute—such a sweet little butterball!" Butterballs are supposed to stay round, aren't they?

"You're Mommy's little dumpling." How many dumplings have you seen with a waistline?

"Daddy's little sugar lump." Aren't sugar lumps square? Will she need to be square to be sweet?

When I adopted my daughter at age seven, she wanted to wear skirts without shoulder straps. "When you get a waistline that reveals some hipbones to hold it up, I'll get you one," I told her. Hipbones? She didn't know she had such things. And they were supposed to be noticeable? Hmmm. I wonder what kind of description she was fed during her early formative years.

When I was small, Daddy said I looked just like his sister— the one who had a small build and never gained weight—that he loved dearly. While I was still very young and active, I was fed a steady diet of: "You can eat anything you want and still stay thin." And Daddy bragged on my figure. Since I loved my daddy a lot, I wanted to continue to please him, so I tried always to look as much like his sister as I could. And he continued to notice the resemblance as long as he lived. Shortly after Daddy died, I gained ten pounds—now that I knew why I had previously kept it off, you can be sure I took charge of the direction of my thoughts from then on. So, when anyone would warn me *you're going to get fat if you eat that*, I would tell myself *that's not true* each time and try to recall childhood words of *you can eat anything you want and still stay thin.*

So—you're fat because that's the way you've been described by the people in your life. But you *stay* fat because you keep repeating to yourself what you've been told … plus a few other things you've made up on the way to now.

My mother stayed fat for years because the family encouraged it. We kids said, "You've got such a nice big lap to sit on," and we'd act very pleased. In fact, we heard Dad use the words "pleasingly plump" often. Dad said her extra weight gave him "more to hug," and he hugged her often. So she didn't lose the extra poundage until she was frightened by her doctor because of all the fat being deposited around an enlarged heart that had a leaky valve. And then she found out he still liked hugging her, even though there was a lot less of her to hug.

And consider for a moment the unconscious motivation of a little boy I'll call Ted. He was told, "The girls won't want to marry you—you'll never get a girl to fall in love with you unless you get that weight off and have a slim figure." This was the warning he heard often during his preteen years when many kids put on a little extra weight just before they enter those rapid growth years. But no one understood that Ted was in love with his mother, and still believed he could grow up and marry her. He never wanted to leave her. So he began eating even more and gained an enormous amount of weight without the least understanding of the reasons why. After all, Mother loved him just the way he was—any way he was. It was Dad and his brothers who nagged about his weight. They were probably just jealous of his close relationship with his mother, he told himself. Dad had criticized Mother about her weight too, but it never did any good. So Ted grew both up and out. He told himself it was hereditary—his mother was fat, too. It couldn't possibly have anything to do with the fondness for chocolate cake and homemade bread that they both shared.

While his brothers became fond of swimming, bike riding, and helping Dad outside, Ted found solace in a book or in front of the TV set. After all, Dad liked them best, he told himself. And if he stayed close to the kitchen, he wouldn't miss any pans that might need licking ... or the smell of hot bread baking in the oven.

And then there was a woman—let's call her Mrs. Bountiful—who secretly feared she would not be able to stay faithful to her husband. She had a real cute figure and heads turned wherever she went. Lots of men flirted with her and even propositioned her whenever they got the chance. It was becoming increasingly difficult for her to say "no."

Like Arnold, she'd also heard, "No one loves a fatty," so on went the pounds until she became so hidden in the mounds of fat that her will power was no longer tested by those would-be pursuers.

But some people never develop will power. They are the ones whose parents give them whatever they ask for, and they never have to wait to have a request fulfilled. If they were never denied anything they wanted as they were growing up, why would they deny themselves anything they want after they're on their own? Habits are formed quite early in life—especially eating habits and food preferences.

And, heaven forbid! Some parents even bribed their little ones into or out of various behaviors with food. So after those children grow into adulthood, whenever they feel blue, they eat. Whenever they've accomplished something special, they eat. Food has become both a solace and a reward, depending upon the associations made early in life between behavior and food. Even an animal can be taught that food follows certain actions. Haven't we all seen people reward a dog for retrieving a ball or doing a trick on command? Haven't we seen circus animals rewarded with a favorite tasty tidbit for each obedient behavior? Think about that for a moment. Are you really being pampered … or controlled? Do you want someone else to hold up the hoop and say "Jump!"?

Yes, there are a great many reasons people become fat—or stay fat. Some associate it with success. During my youth, rich people were often depicted as being fat. If you had money, you could eat anything you wanted; success was measured by the circumference of the waist, especially if you were male.

And other people associated thinness with illness—probably

because those who develop certain types of illnesses waste away rapidly. Whatever the reason, plumpness was considered attractive—the "Twiggy" look was not "in." Thin people were thought to be weaklings … and downright sickly looking. "You need to put some meat on those bones!" kids were told.

When you're very small, you believe that your parents, or those in charge of you, are always right. So a lot of what you are was fed to you so early you may have forgotten what you were told. But by looking at you, I can pretty well guess what *someone* told you!

Feelings about those around you also come into play. If you feel resentment for a person, you will most likely try to be the opposite of what that person wants you to be. I resented the heavier people in my life who told me I was too thin. I figured they were just jealous—after all, my parents, whom I loved, told me I was just right. So you need to do some self-examination of feelings and see how you feel about the people who are describing you.

What parents say can really have an effect—and not only on size. When my daughter was young, her dad told her she would catch cold if she washed her hair when the weather was extra cold. Wasn't that a prediction and a half? So she washed it anyway, and every time she washed it during very cold weather, she promptly caught cold … until she grew up and decided he was wrong.

We eat a little bit too much and what happens—someone says, "Watch out! You're going to get fat." So those who believe it, obligingly do.

Oh yes, beliefs are very important! What do you hold within you as truth? What do you expect out of life?

Some years ago, I met a little old lady who was nearly blind in one eye. During the course of our first conversation, she told me that throughout her growing up years her mother had been blind in one eye—on the same side of the head as this lady's almost blind eye. "All of my life, I wondered if I would become blind in one eye when I was older, too," she revealed, in a lowered, somewhat mysterious tone, as though this was indication of mystical prophetic powers ... of which she herself was more than a little mystified. "And, now, I wonder if I'll also lose the sight in my other eye, since my mother was totally blind by the time she died," the lady continued.

What is it the Bible says about that? "For the thing which I greatly feared is come upon me, and that which I was afraid of is come unto me." (Job 3:25)

As we talked, I learned it was not even a type of blindness that is hereditary. But she had feared it all along—which meant she secretly believed she would be blind, and I couldn't seem to convince her to change her thoughts.

We could all be pretty psychic and "see" into our futures. All we have to do is analyze what we think about all day long. We are what we think ... and expect ... and believe.

A friend and I were discussing what we expected, health-wise, in the future. "I'm going to have arthritis when I'm older," he said.

It was beyond me why this young person would want something like that, so I asked him, "Why do you want to have arthritis?"

The look he gave me suggested I might have grown a second head, and he proceeded to explain to me that he didn't "want" to have it, but his grandparents and all the oldsters of his family developed arthritis when they got older, so he had presumed it was an inevitable part of his getting old. But how much of what we become is hereditary, and how much is expected because of the role models we see around us? I had never associated arthritis with "getting old" since none of the elders in my family had ever had it. So, we ended up having quite a discussion about "getting what one believes one will get if the belief is held long enough."

Listen to the people around you. Listen carefully. They will tell you, without meaning to, what they believe ... what they have created for themselves ... or are in the process of creating. During my travels, I met a woman who told me she had a severe case of asthma that periodically sent her to the hospital. She really wouldn't have had to tell me about it, as she repeated, "I'm holding my breath until...." several times during the next fifteen minutes of our conversation.

You might say it's the old chicken or the egg type situation and speculate as to which came first, but I know we create with our thoughts. That's why my bet is down on the words, following the thoughts, preceding the condition.

Listen to the words used habitually—those repeated over and over again. Just saying, or thinking, something once is very unlikely to create a condition, but repeated over time—while the cells of your body are being replaced—can, and does, bring about whatever you think or say.

When I first became aware of this, I began paying attention to words I used habitually. One word in particular was used quite often: "anxious". "I am *anxious*" had been applied to a variety of statements. And here I had wondered why I was filled with anxiety all the time!

Of course, we all know the word "anxious" can mean desirous of something as well as being worried or distressed. But when I first learned to use the word in my youth, and therefore acquired the habit of using it, the more negative connotation was the only one I knew. So that was the message that was entered into my subconscious memory bank. Later, when I learned it can be used either way, it was like two people with the same initials and last name banking at the same bank. It could become pretty confusing. So when I use the word, my body tenses as though something dreadful is about to happen.

But tension is tension, and too much of it is detrimental to the body. It doesn't make too much difference whether I tensed because I was "anxious" from desire or dread.

Besides saying such things as, "I am *anxious* to go with you" and "I'm *anxious* to hear from you," I also said, "I will be *anxiously* awaiting your return." How about *that* for a prophecy! And, I was right. I was *anxious* almost all the time until I began to pay close attention to my patterns of thought and speech.

And as I did so, I noticed how often I said, "I'm tired of _____." People can fill in that blank with an endless number of words: hot weather, cold weather, this noise, taking care of these kids, his job, those people, cleaning this house, mowing this yard, etc., etc., etc. I had my own endless variety of situations and conditions I attached those words to. Is it any wonder I was tired so much of the time?

Some people use the word "hate" like I used "tired." Are they truly loving people? Or are they filled with anger ... or resentments?

I wonder how many people who said, "You're driving me crazy!" over and over—or that "this" or "that" is driving them crazy—actually ended up having so-called nervous breakdowns. I'll bet, at the very least, many of them ended up using tranquilizers regularly, or had to go into therapy.

And even signs don't say what they mean. Not long ago, I stayed at a RV park. The little house that contained the rooms marked "Ladies" and "Gentlemen" also had a sign stating "For Park Guests Only." Now, who do they think they're kidding? No one there was a *guest.* In fact, I've never stopped for an overnight at one that didn't expect some green to exchange hands. And all over the USA, signs say "Restroom," yet no one *rests* there!

For many years, due to my paralysis, I had a bladder retention problem. The fact is, I spent so many years stopping at every roadside structure that harbored a commode (or hole in the wood) that my husband at that time referred to me as a "Restroom Inspector." When we rode with others, he frequently asked the driver to, "Stop! Billy has to check that restroom."

Using that familiar term caused me some consternation once while spending a summer in Canada. I planned to attend Easter services at the local church. So after confession Saturday evening, I asked the priest if the church had a restroom. "Yes," he said, "come through the side door when you arrive, climb the stairs, and turn to your right." Sunday morning I followed his directions. Upon making the right turn, there stood Father with a big welcoming smile, holding a chair for me to "rest" in while I attended services.

Why do we say things we don't mean even at the time we begin saying them? Force of habit. We hear or read words over and over until they are familiar. We repeat them to ourselves and then to others. They become habit. We use them in first this context and then that context, until, eventually, we aren't even aware that we've used the words at all—much less that they are out of place in the sentences in which we use them.

But remember, that old subconscious mind (your very own internal computer with the life-size print-outs) accepts those words without judging whether you really want to be tired, hateful, crazy, angry, etc. It just latches onto the word, hooks it up with the appropriate feeling and creates for you what you said you wanted.

Just as facial wrinkles and lines show what you've thought about most of your life, your size also shows what you've been thinking about yourself.

Some of you had mothers who said, "Have a second piece of cake, it won't hurt you!" So, sure, you can blame your mother. But, what good does that do you? You're still fat!

You've been spoon-fed this description of yourself that you don't like, so it's their fault! You feel you *need* someone ... or something ... to blame. Okay. Fine. Go ahead and do it and get it over with ... and then forget it, so you can get on with the task at hand—to be thin. It's *your* responsibility—*you're* the one who wants to be thin.

We could analyze all day to see how you got that way, but what's the use? The treatment will still be the same. When you look in the mirror, you know you're doing something wrong, or you'd be the way you want to be. Thin.

Here is an important fact that you need to remember: If no one in your world describes you the way you want to be, then do it yourself. Don't forever sit back and accept descriptions of yourself that you don't want to be. Why let others control your life ... and size? Take charge! Start creating a new you.

According to biologists, some individual cells in the human body live approximately four months.[1] I have heard that within a period of seven years, most of the body has been replaced, cell by cell. Since we continue to replace ourselves with about the same size and shape, we must be using the same pattern of thought.

What kind of pattern is your subconscious mind holding? Let's examine the evidence. The evidence is staring back at you from your mirror. Want to change the pattern you continue to create yourself from? Then read on.

But before we conclude this chapter, let's again go back to Arnold. We looked at some of the many reasons he got fat; now let's examine some of the reasons he's stayed fat so long. For one thing, Arnold always told himself, "I can't run as fast as the other boys, because I'm too heavy—it wouldn't be good for my heart if I did." At other times he said, "I'd probably have a heart attack if I worked as hard as he does, since I'm so much overweight." So now he's justified not being active enough to burn up the extra calories he eats; therefore, he gets even fatter. He also doesn't have to compete—which he really didn't want to do anyway but needed a reason not to. Or so he thought.

And then there's always good old heredity. Learning to like the same fattening foods fat relatives like couldn't possibly have anything to do with it, could it? Even if Arnold hadn't liked

Uncle George so much, he might have decided he would be like him because he's related—besides the fact that everyone said he was like him. Arnold had lots of fat relatives, so he could always blame heredity. After all, if he wanted to be fat and comfortable about it, he needed something to blame it on.

But now he says, "I've *got* to lose weight…," so it has become very important to him in terms of becoming lovable. Remember, he has been told, "No one loves a fatty," and he believes that. Besides, news reports have been released recently about the dangers of an earlier death from being overweight, so now he has added incentive to get that weight down.

But, not only has Arnold created his past and his present, he has begun to create his future with his thoughts—"…it's going to be hard."

It just couldn't be easy, right?

Wrong! Will someone please give him a copy of this book?

Chapter Three

What Tense Do You Use?

Upon further examination of Arnold's statement, we find he has used future tense in both his inner and outer language. Aloud, he said, "I'm going to lose this weight," and to himself, he said, "…it's going to be hard." Both are in the future, and the future never comes.

I imagine we have all heard about the old pencil test of holding a pencil between thumb and index finger while saying, "I'm going to drop this pencil." You don't drop it until you decide to do so "now." It's kind of like the beginning of a race. The race is going to start as soon as someone shouts "Go!"— meaning right *now*. All of the things we are going to do never get done until we put them in the "now."

So ... another important concept: In order to change your reality—that which is real for you—you must change your internal speech patterns and your description of yourself ... and it has to be in the present tense.

Communication with yourself is even more important than your communication with other people. If Arnold wants to be thin, he will have to change how he describes himself—first to himself ... and then to others.

It's as easy as that. He is what he is because he was told how he was, and would be, first by others and then by himself. The planet is full of things created by thought. Someone had an idea—a thought, then came the creation of that thought. When things need to be done over—refurbished—there must be a new idea of that change before the deed is even started.

So now, to change *yourself*, change what you tell *yourself* about *yourself*. Create a new you, so to speak. But stay away from the negative. What good would it do if you were in the process of recovering a chair in green, to say, "I don't want it brown anymore; I want it to be green!"? That was the thought you had that caused you to decide to change it in the first place—someday. But now you are busy recovering it, so you say, "I am recovering this chair in green." Hear that word "am"? Put your thoughts into the present—the *now*.

"I *am* thin."

No? You say you can't say you are when you're not?

"I cannot tell a lie," you say.

Really? You always tell the truth about yourself? I wonder just how many people *always* do.

Why, I remember hearing people say, "I'm a monkey's uncle." Did one of their siblings actually mate with a monkey?

Someone enters the room. Anyone already there might give the greeting, "What do you know?" "Nothing," is the reply. Want to bet?

Ever hear a politician say, "This honor leaves me speechless," and leave it at that?

When you hear someone say, "I worked my fingers to the bone today," do you look to see how much bone is exposed?

Someone else says, "I am completely out of breath." Wonder how he was able to make the statement.

"My feet are killing me!" Does she have gangrene?

"I'm bored to death." Should we order flowers?

"My head is splitting." Hold everything! My camera's in the next room.

A young fellow, disgusted with himself because he didn't know how to accomplish a task, suddenly found out it was really quite simple and was heard to say, "I'm a son of a bitch." Come on now! Let's not drag Mama into this—or maybe he meant he came from a doggie litter.

And *you* might even have said, "I am frozen!" when you came in from the freezing weather, but I'll bet you were just cold—and probably that was only skin deep. I doubt your temperature had dropped very much.

Point accepted? Now let me tell you a not-so-well-kept secret. You are actually a spirit living in a fat bodysuit. Is a spirit fat or thin? Are you sure? Well, if you're not sure, then your spirit could just as well be thin as fat, and I say it is thin. You've said all along, "I am fat," and you couldn't even see your real self when you looked into your mirror. So go ahead and try it my way. Say, "I am thin." Say it to yourself often. Believe it, because it's true. *You are thin.* You just have some unneeded shrouding that you will shed like an old outdated suit of clothes as soon as you accept this principle.

In the beginning, if you just simply cannot say, "I am thin," then say, "I am thinner as I shed these pounds," or "My body is a little thinner each day; I am thinner than I was yesterday." Just remember that whatever you want to have happen, put it in the "now."

It is ... I am ... I have ... I believe....

Whatever you want out of life, make a *Positive Now Statement*—a *PNS*. It can be made mentally or orally—preferably both—but make it *NOW*.

Stop worrying about what you have to give up or what you don't want. In fact, stop worrying! You attract to you what you resist. Instead of saying, "I don't want to be fat," or "I have to stop eating this or that," say, "I am thinner" or "I know carrots are good for my eyes and skin, so I like them."

Analyze your thoughts and manner of using words, both orally and silently. Clean up your act! Your way of communicating with yourself and others is the first thing that must be changed in order to change yourself and your reality. It's worth all the effort you can possibly put into it. Replace all negative words with positive ones. Change the way you think about yourself—the way you describe yourself.

The "T" in F.A.T. stands for *Thought*. Thought created the extra padding you carry around with you, and thought can change that which thought has created.

Lay out a new pattern over the old material on your cutting board, and before long, you'll see a sleek new suit of clothes covering the spirit smiling back from your mirror.

Chapter Four

Making the Right Decision

How many of you have dieted and lost weight only to gain it all back, plus maybe a little more? Did you then go on another diet ... lose it again ... gain it back ... lose ... gain ... lose ... gain?

If so, then perhaps your decision was "to lose weight" rather than "to be thin." When you make a decision "to lose weight," you *have* to gain it back so you can "lose" it! Therefore, making the right decision is extremely important. The right decision leads to proper actions.

So ... if you have been a gain-again, lose-again person, change your decision to "be thin and stay that way." See why it is necessary to think of yourself as already thin? When you only see yourself as a person "losing weight," you may be doomed to repeat the process for the rest of your life. Anything I can say to help put the idea of already being thin into your mind is worth every effort to convince you. How quickly we all are to put thoughts such as "I am suffocating" immediately into our minds when the room becomes just a little stuffy. Yes, we can put *other* concepts that obviously aren't true at the time into the "now," but feel we can't say, "I am thin" unless we can actually see the evidence of that fact. Yet, you *are* thin under there somewhere; you just have layers and layers of cells trying to hide you. It's kind of like having on a dress underneath a big bulky overcoat.

Would you say the dress isn't there because it isn't showing?

Okay now, make a brand new decision "to be thin," and at every opportunity, tell yourself, "I *am* thin."

How long will it take after the decision is made? Well, that will depend upon your reasons for wanting to be thin. Do you want to be thin because an acquaintance or someone in your family wants you to be thin? What would happen if you later met someone who thought you would look better heavier? You can't please everyone—so forget what "they" want you to be. Be what *you* want to be. Don't let other people control your weight; control it yourself.

So what do *you* want: "to be, or not to be"[2] thin? Are you pleased with what you see when you look into your mirror? Take off all your clothes and watch yourself as you turn slowly around. Like what you see? Then stay that way. No incentive there.

But what if you look at yourself and say, "Ugh! Disgustingly fat?" That's a beginning and possible mover toward getting something done about it. Another motivator is when one decides, as did Arnold, that someone won't love you unless you're thin—someone besides yourself, that is.

While I was at the university studying to become a counselor, one of my professors told the class about someone who had been extremely heavy for many years. Then she fell for a man who seemed to prefer slimmer women. Well, she dropped those pounds so fast one would have thought her very life depended upon it! The race was on, and the trophy was marriage. With that incentive, the excess fatty tissue was rapidly reduced to: "You're looking great!" But after she settled smugly into her new conjugal life, the pounds slowly crept right back into place.

Her decision had not been "to be thin"; it was "to get a man." And she got him!

Overeating is a lot like other bad habits—such as smoking. Smoking came natural for me. My mother and father both smoked. My older brother smoked. Then my husband … my friends. So I just naturally drifted into the habit. After all, I breathed it everyday … everywhere … and I liked the smell of smoke. No one told me of the risks involved; back then, no one seemed to know there were any. No one told me how hard it would be to quit—I never looked that far down the road. But when the evidence began mounting that spoke of the dangers of the habit, I tried to quit … several times, but it just seemed too difficult. Each time I'd quit, I'd started right back up again, before long. My decision had been "to quit smoking" rather than "to be a nonsmoker," and my motivators were not sufficiently strong. *Others* were saying I *should* quit for "other" peoples' reasons. But eventually I had a reason of my own to break the habit. It was the best reason of all—the strongest motivator: Life preservation.

For some time, I had been extremely tired—exhausted—but I just couldn't put a label on exactly what was causing it. Maybe it was "tired blood"—so I tried an iron tonic. It didn't help. I got more rest, but I only became even more tired. My physical examination that year hadn't turned up any new discoveries, but I remained so tired I could barely get my housework done. Just sweeping the floor required several sit-downs.

Then one morning, I happened to notice my heart was racing way over 100 beats per minute, and I had done nothing more strenuous than pour myself a cup of coffee and light my first cigarette of the day. My heart was beating as though I had just run a race, and I was as bone-weary tired as if I had, indeed, been trying to win the longest marathon.

What could be causing it?

Next morning, I checked my pulse as soon as I got up. Normal. Lit a cigarette, zoom—off to the race! After the second cigarette, it was speeding so fast one would think I had a nest of angry hornets after me—it was no wonder I was tired. So I vowed not to smoke the next morning and see what happened.

Maybe it was just coincidence. Or maybe it was my morning coffee I always drank with the first cigarette. Surely it couldn't be tobacco that caused the acceleration in my pulse rate, because the other times I'd temporarily given up the leaf, I'd not noticed any change in my health at all. *Everyone* had said I would, but I hadn't. So it wasn't long before I'd light up again, smug in the conviction that "everyone" was wrong.

Well, you guessed it. My earlier attempts to stop smoking had not been successful because I hadn't yet developed an allergic reaction to tobacco. I had been younger and healthier and couldn't feel the difference when I refrained from the habit. But now I was definitely in desperate need of energy. And my heart beat did not increase the next day when I didn't light up. It wasn't the coffee. Before long, my energy level picked up, and I could *feel* the delightful difference, so I joined the ranks of the permanently reformed. I became a nonsmoker; now that I knew my very life depended upon it. And "to be, or not to be"[3] alive is the strongest of all motivators for change.

The best stimulus for losing weight also seems to be health; it's more apt to stay off when you can actually *feel* the benefits as well as see them. And the more urgent the reason, the faster it comes off, too. Most people don't want to die. A prognosis of "You won't live much longer unless you get that weight off" seems to be a dandy motivator!

I recall my mother's doctor telling her just that. Mother had gradually added pound after pound until she was ashamed to be seen in public and began shying away from all but the most pressing engagements. Finally her doctor just flat out told her it was an "either ... or" situation. You never saw anyone get more serious about losing weight! Mother supplied me with enough material for essay after essay in my high school English classes during the next several semesters. Mother didn't think her weight loss program (and antics) was as funny as I did, though, and she put a stop to my using her for classroom material after coming across one of my essays I'd prepared for the next day's class.

I also have a friend who found out her weight was causing her problems similar to the ones I experienced from smoking. She moved into a brand new house with a staircase between the main floor and her basement sewing and recreation rooms. It got so she could barely drag herself up and down the stairs. Not having had stairs to climb in her former house, she had not been previously aware of the effect her added pounds were having on her health. So she adopted a strict dietary program, lost about a hundred pounds and was absolutely thrilled with the difference in both her energy level and how quickly and easily she could go up and down those stairs. "I don't think my heart could have taken too many more years of the strain of carrying all that weight around," she confided, and then stated firmly, "And I'm never going to gain it back."

So, examine your reasons why you want to be thin and discover whether your motivators are strong enough—or do you just want to please someone else? Arnold didn't want to be thin for himself, or he probably would have been thin all along—even before he met Mary. He secretly wishes Mary would love him even though he *is* fat, but he doesn't believe she will. Since he isn't planning to lose it for himself—but only so Mary will love him—he may, indeed, find the losing "hard" to do.

No one loses for someone else's reasons—unless out of fear. That's not a good reason, however, because just as soon as the source of fear is gone, the weight goes right back up.

One day, I asked my first husband to put a new hole in my old leather belt. "What's the matter—getting too fat?" He just naturally assumed people's weight change is always up, and he definitely did not want *me* to get heavy. Why, when we were just newlyweds, he threatened to divorce me if I ever got heavy. Fact is, he had such a strong aversion to fat that he stayed so thin himself that, were he to lose any more weight, he'd have had to wear weighted shoes to prevent a strong wind from sending him into orbit. And the snide remarks, when weight was mentioned, were calculated to frighten me into instant watchfulness.

"No," I replied, "it needs to be an inch smaller." I don't need, or want, a weight watchdog. I have my very own set of motivators that has kept me wearing the same size ever since I was sixteen years old. Besides having pride in my looks and respect for my body, I also *need* to stay on the lighter side of life. Although I have retrained my body so I can walk again, walking has been difficult for me ever since the accident and it would be impossible if I became heavy-footed. So I am self-motivated—I don't work on the fear-of-others principle.

There are many hidden problems that prevent people from making that "be thin" decision or sticking to it after it has been made. One woman stays fat because of the nagging insistence of her mate that she be thin. There is an inner resentment between them that has never been resolved.

And Nancy, who had been heavy as a child and only attracted her mate after a successful "weight loss" program, is getting heavy again because she is fearful that her husband doesn't *really* love her—just her body. So she feels she needs to gain weight in order to prove, once and for all to herself, that he loves *her* regardless of size. Or is she just using him as a reason to go back to the old way of eating? Well, even if she does somehow prove to herself whether he loves her or not, she may relapse into eating habits that will take even more effort to change by that time.

Then too, there are those who find it impossible to lose weight, because, even though they *want* to, they are giving in to someone else's wishes. They are letting someone else's insecurities insert unwanted programs into their "computers"— putting thoughts into their heads that prevent them from making a clear, definite "be thin" decision. They are allowing others to have squatter's rights where they don't belong. Oh, not that the other person is always *aware* of that process—but that doesn't change the fact that it is being allowed to happen.

One man I know encourages his wife to stay fat because that way he feels he won't lose her to another. It's his insurance that she won't stray. His own lack of self-confidence keeps him bringing home candy in the name of "love" and urging her to eat a little more because he likes her on the plump side. If she only knew the underlying motivator!

Be forewarned that others may be working in opposition to your wish to be thin. Being aware is half the battle when it comes to a full-scale war of wills.

Frankly, I don't like to let others make my decisions for me—I had enough of that as a child. I don't want others to have power over me; as an adult, I make my own decisions. I want my thoughts to be my own. Don't let other people tell you what to think. Decide for yourself what you want to think about and then do it. When you catch yourself thinking about things you've heard others say, stop and check it out. See if it needs to be changed. Decide to think about how good you feel, how much less you weigh, how thin you are, your decision to be thin. Be glad you've discovered the way to change your life—because you have by the time you've read this book.

Don't just blindly follow another's lead, especially a selfish one like the candy man's. Take off your blinders and look at those greener fields on either side of the path you are presently on—the thin "you," who is healthier, happier, and more fulfilled, is right there within easy reach.

The decision to take control of your thoughts comes first. Desire only comes after you think about a thing—emotion follows thought. So *decide* what you will think about consciously. Don't just let ideas and thoughts that conflict with being thin arise from your subconscious mind—those thoughts that you have previously allowed to take up residence there— and habitually spend time thinking about. Break the old pattern. Write down all the things you want to be and think about them instead.

Before anything really happens, there must be a decision made. If you want to be thin, then you will need to make a decision to be thin. But if you don't change your internal and external way of communication, then you have *not* made a new decision.

You say you *have* made a "thin" decision? And you've tried diet after diet to no avail? Well sure, and you could go on buying diet book after diet book; you could go on one diet for a while and then another for the rest of your life. Yes, the authors of those books were just the size you wanted to be—and with high hopes, as you happily purchased each book, you assumed that in no time at all you'd look just like the latest model of perfection. But then, after all the tortures of trying to follow the prescribed program, you looked into your mirror and could by no stretch of the imagination see a "model of perfection" staring back at you.

What went wrong? We both know something didn't work out, or you wouldn't be reading this book.

The problem lies in incentive ... or lack of a strong one. The authors of the books you bought had a stronger incentive to be thin than you had. Most of them had profit in mind. A female movie star stays slim because her figure is the profit maker, along with acting ability. Strong incentive! Their living depends on it. I once knew a girl who taught dancing and worked as exercise leader for a health spa. She worried if she gained five pounds—it could affect her ability to earn her living. And there was the bonus of admiring looks and comments if she kept her weight down.

So examine your incentives—your motivators. Are they strong? Have you made a clear-cut decision to be thin? If you have, then you are now ready to proceed with the active part of being thin; the "A" in F.A.T. stands for *Action*.

Now, don't let that word "action" scare you off. My kind of action isn't a strenuous workout, so read on. Being thin depends more on mental processes than on physical ability.

PART TWO

Act Thin

Chapter Five

Make Moving Choices

Action means: (1) Get Started, and (2) move. To be thin, we need both. A decision has not really been made unless we follow through and put it into action. Faith in our ability to accomplish something is demonstrated by acting as though we have it already. So you must start doing something you will do when you arrive at the weight you wish to be. Act like whatever you want to be. Why do you want to be thin? Go ahead and *do* whatever you say you will do when you're at your proper weight—only in more moderation.

So, now that you have made your decision to be thin and have started monitoring your speech and thoughts, it is time to choose a role model. A role model is someone you place in the position of one you desire to be like. We all have role models whether we consciously choose them or not. After watching Mama feed baby brother or sister, little girls may practice on their dolls; they are using Mama as a role model to become a mother. Or, in this day of women's liberation, it could be Dad they watch at work in order to become a truck driver or a mechanic. Some child, aspiring to become a movie star, big-time singer, or dancer, may spend hours in a theater or in front of the TV set watching the one they emulate. Whatever we want to be, we watch those who do it; we want to act like them and look like them.

Okay. You want to be thin, so pick out someone to play the role of *The Thin Person* for you. This person should have a figure like you'd like to show the world. Don't choose a picture from a magazine. Choose someone you know, preferably, or someone whose day-to-day actions you observe fairly often. If you watch the behavior of The Thin Person, you will begin to notice certain movements that differ from yours. Watch The Thin Person you've chosen carefully. Analyze your model's way of walking, moving, and living. Notice any behaviors different from yours? Does that person walk faster? Climb stairs instead of taking the elevator? Get up and down during each commercial while watching TV? Enjoy a sport such as swimming or bike riding? Dance? Sleep less?

If you want to emerge from your cocoon as the beautifully slim you, then choose just one behavior in which *you* do not engage on a regular basis and perform it until it becomes a part of your lifestyle. Choose any one you please. It doesn't have to be a difficult movement. In fact, if you are extremely overweight or have medical problems, please check with your doctor before attempting any strenuous physical movements. At first, just choose an easy-to-do action that your role model uses and you don't.

Too many of you must have thought that old saying, "If you don't use it, you lose it," applied to fat as well as muscles; but, I hope by now you've already discovered this fallacy. You *move* it to remove it.

Just for a moment, think about what a farmer does when he wants to fatten up his livestock for market. He confines them to close quarters in order to keep exercise to a minimum. The cattle are corralled; the pigs are penned. Exercise would burn up calories from the extra feed he plans to give them. Feed is expensive and time is important. He wants to fatten them in the shortest period of time at the least expense. The more they weigh, the more he makes. No exercise, plus more feed, equals fat animals.

Now, apply that principle—only in reverse. Any movement performed regularly that you don't already make will use more calories than you burn at present. And we all know what calories are. They're those little units of energy that we burn up in daily living or store away as fat for future use ... and store ... and store ... and store (just like the cattle and the pigs) if we don't *use* them as we ingest them. But there will be more about that subject in the next chapter. Right now, we're concerned with behaviors other than eating.

In my youth, I was the thinnest member of my immediate family. There were several differences in my habits and those of the heavier members—some deliberately chosen, some not. Take mealtimes, for instance. As soon as each meal ended, I was told to clear the table and do the dishes while Mother poured herself a cup of coffee with added calories and retired to her living room easy chair. The others dispersed to their favorite resting places to digest their food. My sister ate so slowly that you could say she was following suit as she remained seated two or three times as long as the others. I recall hearing a neighbor say, "It doesn't matter how long it takes her to eat; she'll get more good out of her food that way." We all know one shouldn't exercise strenuously for twenty minutes following a big meal, but if one rests a lot longer than that after every meal, more of it is going to be stored. Years later, after we were all grown and had scattered to various places, Mother said, "I wonder if making you jump right up from the table and stay busy for thirty minutes or so had anything to do with your staying thinner?"

Yes, habits are formed early. I still clear the table and do the dishes right after meals.

Some of you who are overweight may, of course, do the same. If so, then look further; maybe it's your sleep habits. That was another difference in our family. Mother stayed up late, slept late, and nearly always took a nap. All in all, she usually racked up ten or more hours out of twenty-four. My sister and older brother slept later than I did and moved less during sleep. My sister and I slept together in a big double bed for years, and I know she slept much sounder than I did, which accounted for the less nighttime movement. I was awake long after she went to sleep, and I was up and out before anyone else, except Dad.

Okay, so you can't do anything about how much you move or don't move during sleep, but you can choose how much *time* you sleep.

Some time ago, scientists discovered that a prolonged period spent lying prone slows the circulation to the point of possible danger. There is more chance of a circulatory disorder; there is more loss of calcium.[4] It was recommended that one sleep no longer than seven or eight hours at a time. A short nap in the afternoon was advised if more rest or sleep was needed. Actually, a ten or fifteen minute siesta halfway through one's awake time seems to renew vigor and promote alertness. However, long afternoon naps—especially those over an hour long—work just the opposite. One may feel more tired and sluggish from too much sleep, either night or day.

And less sleep gives more time for action—more chances to burn calories. If you sleep more than eight hours, set your alarm and get up earlier. I used those early morning hours to work in the garden before the sun had a chance to heat up the Earth. And I have a friend who is conscious of what part activity plays in weight control; she finds getting up earlier than her family gives her time to do odd jobs like wiping fingerprints off appliances, clearing away cobwebs, or weeding the flower beds. Before becoming activity conscious, when she happened to wake up early, she would spend mornings watching the news or reading with a cup of coffee at hand. Now, if she does decide to watch the news, she folds clothes or in some other way stays busy.

I'm sure you can find some action you could do with an

extra hour or so that you don't do now. How about walking to work or school? Even if you only sleep eight hours now, after you practice the relaxation techniques found later on in this book, you may only need seven. Plan an activity for the extra time. Don't just sit and read or watch TV.

Speaking of TV—cut out part of your viewing time. How about one hour less while you take a walk instead? Practice getting up during each commercial and walking around the room. Get a drink of water ... or water a plant ... anything that takes movement.

Have you ever noticed the difference in people as they watch TV? Some sit extremely still; others move some part of their anatomy. Several extra heavy people I know sit so still one wonders how they stay awake or why their legs don't go numb. Maybe they do. But most of the thinner people tap a toe or move in some way quite often.

Sometimes I crochet while listening to TV. If I get really interested in making something rather large, I lose five or ten pounds in a couple of weeks. Same thing happens when I type the manuscript for a new book because it's in addition to my usual activity.

And don't listen to those people who give out advice on how to save steps and save your energy! Economy of movement might increase efficiency on the job, but at home it just increases weight. I purposely place things I know I'll want often just out of reach, so I'll have to get up and down more. It all depends on which is more important for you—time or weight.

As you stand while stirring something on the stove or outside watering the lawn, move some part of you besides the hand holding the implement of work. I recall watching Mother hit her hips with the heel or her free hand as she stood cooking the evening meals; the fat would jiggle like two cats in a jitterbug contest. That was just one of the many tactics she employed when she really got serious about being her ideal weight.

But maybe you know a thin person who isn't very active and never seems to move. Ever think that person may have a problem—health, depression—or maybe eats a lot less than you'd like to? There are always exceptions, but we're talking about normal, average people here—like most of you.

So, after you've chosen an activity or behavior of your role model that you wish to imitate, then practice, practice, practice. Repeat that movement until it becomes a habit. Then pick out another one. Practice until it, too, becomes part of your lifestyle. Then choose another. Practice. Keep repeating the process until you become an active person. Of course, don't emulate your chosen one to the point of being a carbon copy. But the more active you become, the easier it will be to be a thin person for the rest of your life. More action produces more energy, too. The more you do, the more you *can* do.

What's that you say? Those people just move a lot because they're nervous? Some do, some don't. Movement to some people is enjoyable. It's torture for them to have to sit still for long periods of time, although they can when they so choose. You can learn (and will, later in this book) how to relax the parts of your body that are not currently moving. It's all in learning how. And when relaxed people move, the movement is quite different from that of tense people.

Besides the movement you choose in imitation of The Thin Person, there are two behaviors I want you to do. First, if you can walk, walk after meals. It has been determined that more weight is lost if you walk after a meal than before one.[5] Be sure to wait twenty minutes, but no longer than thirty minutes after eating. If you're not in the habit of walking, start slow and build up. Five minutes even once a day is five minutes more than before you started. After about a week you should be accustomed to that much, so increase it to ten minutes. Continue increasing the time until you walk twenty minutes once a day ... then perhaps even twice a day.

Walk briskly! Don't carry anything on one arm or on one shoulder. If you tote something with you, put it on your back. Some people carry something, like a pound can of vegetables in each hand, and they swing their arms back and forth as they walk. This helps tone upper body muscles while helping to lose weight.

Second, start massaging that fat! Every time you are idle for any reason, grab a handful and knead it, roll it, lightly slap it, or squeeze it gently. Move it in any manner you choose, but don't bruise the flesh. You don't need to be black and blue in order to work it off. If you bruise, you're going after that fat too hard. After massaging a few minutes in one spot, move to another.

Lots of women have lumpy fat—cellulite—especially on their thighs and hips. These lumps are a mixture of fat, water, and waste materials. They need to be broken up and flushed out of the body, just like all of the other waste products. They are the results of the wrong diet, an accumulation of chemical and poisonous matter, and not enough circulation (movement) in the areas in which they are deposited. Lightly squeeze a handful of fat and see if it looks lumpy. If it does, you have cellulite! The quickest way to remove it is to *move* it—and not only by exercising. It needs to be manually moved ... and moved ... until it is gone.

And you get a bonus! Using your arms and hands to work that fat helps burn calories, so you lose weight that much faster, besides having a smaller body by the time you shed the outer coat. So, work on that fat while you sit reading, watching TV, talking, or writing. One hand is often free and has nothing to do. Give it a job! Make massaging yourself a habit. The increased circulation helps in more ways than one.

Now you're on your way to becoming an active person. Say this to yourself often: "I am an active person." Active people are thinner and healthier. Healthier people are happier. So you could say, "I am a thin, happy, active person."

People who think of themselves as thin find behaving as a thin person easy to do. Therefore, if you have any difficulty with becoming more active—if you keep making excuses for not changing your behavior, walking more, moving more, working off that fat—then go back to square one. That thin decision has to be made first. It all begins with thought. *Action* follows thought. You think of something you want to do, and then you do it.

There is never a better time to start than right now—so get a *move* on! Think thin—act thin!

Chapter Six

Respect Your Body

Do you ever get the feeling that this is a crazy mixed-up world? On the one hand, we are told to keep our weight down and eat lightly. One may even hear those dreaded words "Go on a diet!" and the very next minute the TV blares, "Eat this food—it's delicious!" "Drink this beverage!" We are truly saturated with food commercials.

Everywhere we go, food is served or talked about. "What's your favorite recipe?" "Henry's serves the most delightful meals; you simply *must* go there!" "Let's get together and go out for supper."

It just seems like *everything* is celebrated with food, or *no* food, like the fast days we observed just before feast days when I was a kid. That certainly got our minds focused on food.

There are birthday cakes, wedding cakes, the Easter ham and colored eggs, Thanksgiving turkey with all the trimmings, pumpkin pie, Christmas fruitcake, Halloween candy, and Valentine's Day chocolates. There are ice cream socials, the funeral dinner, you-all-come-and-bring-a-dish, an apple for the teacher, a hot fudge sundae for your favorite gal, a politician's fund-raising dinner at X number of dollars a plate, etc., etc., etc. We use food to bribe, appease, entertain, entice, and gain favor—as well as just because we like it.

Yes, we are in the habit of using food for every imaginable

event and celebration all around the world. No wonder it's so hard to get one's mind off food when it becomes necessary to exercise some control.

Just for a moment, think about the five functions we must perform in order to live: sleep, eat, drink, breathe, and eliminate. We breathe in front of the whole world, and we'll drink with almost anyone. Eating is something we do because we have to, but we are expected to eat with others and in front of all who happen to be nearby. We also need to sleep, but we don't ask our friends to join us in bed in order to celebrate events. It must be considered a step higher on the hierarchy of necessities; sleeping together is reserved for marriage partners and lovers. Guess which function that leaves for the pinnacle of the order.

Besides being a necessity, we *enjoy* eating, but for the sake of our health and size we need to learn all we can about the role food plays in our lives. How long we live, and the degree to which we will enjoy our lives, depends partly upon our knowledge of nutrition—that includes the caloric content of what we eat and drink. If you don't want to learn about food values and at least an approximate count of the calories you use and take in, then you will just have to depend on luck.

Are you lucky?

Check back over your life—no one knows better than you. Do you want to trust something as important as your health to luck?

But you're not much overweight? Well, then maybe your metabolism has just slowed down, if you used to be slim … way back when.

Exercise speeds up the metabolism—the rate at which you burn calories for energy. Perhaps you've dropped an activity you used to do? Pick it back up, or start walking more.

Not obese—just not shaped right? Again, exercise is needed. That part of you that is out-of shape needs to be moved more.

Here's a rule-of-thumb tidbit often used for all you extra heavy heavies: Subtract two years from your life for each inch your waist measurement exceeds your chest measurement.

Does that make you want to go on a diet immediately ... again? Or how about joining a lose-weight organization? Do you know why they usually work—temporarily? Fear principle! You're afraid to go back next week weighing more—you'll lose face in front of the others. There is also the support of others cheering you on. Attention for losing now ... instead of for gaining. But, do you plan to stay with the organization for the rest of your life? Or do you plan to take diet pills the rest of your life? Oh, there are lots of other plans and diets for losing weight, but are they what you want to *do* for the rest of your life?

Withdraw from the plan, diet, group, pills, etc., and back up goes that weight—until you learn to take responsibility for your size and your life.

Sure, you have been misled, misguided, taught to eat the wrong foods—but it's *you* who now wants to lose that weight, live a more productive life, and feel better! So it's *you* who will have to take *Overweight* by the horns and bulldog that critter down.

Yes, someone else might have gotten you started on this merry-go-round—we often take the path of least resistance—but that fact won't make you any slimmer. No siree! The only way to get off the merry-go-round—the diet syndrome (lose it until one can brag about the loss. After no one comments about the losing of it, or it becomes "old hat," or you get to where you wanted to be, you relax and gain it back again) is to take responsibility for yourself, your thoughts, your size and your eating habits. If you had to starve to get it off, you wouldn't dare stay on a starvation diet forever unless you want to become a *real* skeleton, so you have to start eating again. Even if the plan was just a particular diet, who wants to eat the same thing, or follow a plan, forever?

This isn't a health book; it's a how-to-be-thin book.

Otherwise, we'd get into the nitty-gritty of dyes, chemicals, preservatives, etc., in food and drink that are detrimental to your health and may shorten your life just as surely as being overweight does.

Do you recall the warning "When in doubt, throw it out" concerning foods that might be spoiled or contaminated? To my way of thinking, this should be applicable to controversial chemicals in both food and drink, too. If you don't know what's in it, don't eat or drink it.

There are two ways of being thin: thin and healthy; thin and unhealthy. To be healthy, we must focus on nutrition. As the saying goes: "We are what we eat."

But this isn't a complete treatise on nutrition—we'd need a *huge* book … or many volumes! No, this is just a chapter to open your eyes and help you become aware of the role food plays in your life. Later, I'm sure you will want to read more on the subject from other sources.

Actually, what I want to issue here is a learner's permit. Think of yourself as a beginner who needs to learn enough to make wiser choices for your body. What we eat and what we drink are for the purpose of nourishing the body. That's it. That's the beginning. You already knew that, didn't you? But, do you think about it *every time* you put food or drink into your mouth?

Here are a few basic facts that everyone who is interested in both health and size needs to be aware of. Air is our most important requirement, but no one has to tell you to breathe. It just comes naturally.

Next to air, water is the most essential nutrient our bodies require, but unlike air, we often have to be told to drink it. Doesn't that seem odd, since we are mostly made out of water? Why, before taking our places in this world—with a scream of protest—we spent approximately nine months in a swimming pool. The average adult is composed of up to sixty percent water.[6] It is absolutely essential, for our very lives, that we water-dependent creatures replace regularly the water we lose in just ordinary, everyday, staying-alive living.

Water is necessary for the regulation of body temperature and digestion—to carry nutrients to cells and to take wastes from them. What would your blood be without water? You could live much longer without food than without water; it is a part of every cell in your body. Yet we lose water in perspiration and other bodily processes, an amount that must be replaced.

Now that we've established its importance to you, how about making sure you drink your six to eight glasses of water a day as many doctors recommend? Some of what we need is obtained from our food, and of course, lots of other liquids contain water—but they may have calories, or chemicals, or unhealthy substances. Trying to fill your requirement for water with other beverages may supply you with either an overabundance of calories or a toxic supply of alcohol, chemicals, caffeine, etc. Even some water has substances detrimental to health, too. My family uses a filter system on the faucet to remove chlorine and pesticides from our drinking water.

We used to say, "Water is nonfattening—and it's free!" Well, it's not free anymore, generally, but it's cheaper than other liquids; it's still nonfattening ... and it can help fill the stomach. Many are the times I've felt "hungry" and quickly drank a glass of water instead of eating something. It's also helpful to drink a glass of water *before* meals to get a head start on filling the stomach.

When I was a kid, I was told I should drink water, but no one said why. So I figured I got plenty out of what I ate and drank otherwise. I had problems with bladder infections, and later, water retention. Still, no one put sufficient emphasis on drinking water. By the time I finally found out how necessary it is for every bodily function—and for moisturizing the skin to delay the wrinkling process—I had to change half-a-lifetime habit of only drinking perhaps one glass of water a day. Actually, I was using a six-ounce juice glass for water and only filling it as full as necessary in order to swallow whatever supplements I felt were necessary twice a day.

First thing I did was switch to a ten-ounce glass. Second was to keep the glass close to a calendar on which I made a mark each time I drank a glassful of water. Seeing how few marks there were some days encouraged me to drink more. On the days I did drink more, I noticed less water retention and better elimination—both bladder and bowel action was improved. Too much salt plays a big part in water retention for most people, but I did find I could use a little more providing I drank plenty of water. For yourself, always check with your doctor concerning salt and its effect on blood pressure. If there is a water retention problem, usually a low or no-salt diet is recommended.

There are so many *ifs, ands,* and *buts* attached to how much salt is needed by each individual that we are not going to get into that subject here. Salt (sodium) is necessary in varying amounts dependent upon various factors. But since it is present in so much of what we eat, there is usually more need to limit it than to add it.

But let's go back to the subject of water.

Those of you who like to lie out in the sun to bake, think about what happens to wet clothes hung on a line in the sun: the moisture is quickly gone and they become *very* dry. Then think about the elastic in clothes placed in a hot dryer. They lose their elasticity after who-knows-how-few times, right? Do you want your skin to dry out and lose its ability to bounce back—be elastic? The result of lots of sunbathing is dry, wrinkly skin in the-who-knows-how-long-from-now future.

Back when my mother-in-law was my age, she went to a doctor with two problems: a painful knee and constipation. One look at her and he could easily see she would have a lot less problem with her knee if she lost weight; she was quite a bit heavier than was good for her. For both problems he recommended more fiber and eight glasses of water a day. We all know that if you add lots of water to dry fiber (like bran) you get more bulk. Bulk fills the stomach without many calories, and lots of bulk moves waste matter through the intestines more efficiently. More water also fills the tummy and softens the feces.

Right after leaving the doctor's office, she stopped by to tell me what he said. "That fool doctor told me to drink eight glasses of water a day. Why, if I did that I wouldn't be able to eat a thing—I'd be too full!"

He hadn't explained "why"—just said "do it." Of course, she hadn't asked "why" either—that was back when so many felt intimidated by doctors. She certainly did, anyway, at least while she was in his office. Too many of her generation failed to ask questions of those they placed in superior positions. While they were growing up, questions asked of parents often got the response, "Just because I said so!" When that generation left home, they shifted the parental role to doctors.

While we have a little bit of attention focused on elimination, I want to mention the use of laxatives. Laxatives can bring about weight-loss when used regularly—or in excessive doses—but the health of the one using them is affected if they become a habit. It is quite easy to become dependent on them.

When my mother was in her teens, she spent some weeks away from home and Mother. She stayed with her paternal grandmother, who plied her with all sorts of sweets and fattening foods in order to make a favorable impression on the not-often-seen granddaughter. By the time she returned home, my mother had gained twenty pounds of extra weight. Not realizing the risks involved in using laxatives, her mother gave her huge doses of a purgative that kept her on the run until the full twenty pounds was lost. After that, laxatives were given often—anytime she overate or over-gained.

Yes, Mother quickly lost the weight, but she also lost nutrients—both in the food that was being flushed out of the body before what was needed could be absorbed, and in water. Later she came down with rheumatic fever, and she was down for a very long time. When she got out of bed, she had to use crutches and learn to walk all over again. A leaky heart valve was the result of that episode.

One is less likely to be able to fight off infections when nutrients are flushed out on a regular basis, and with the regular use of laxatives, one cannot determine whether enough water and fiber is being taken in. It is usually recommended that fiber, along with enough water to soften the bulk, should be increased until the bowels move regularly and are of a proper consistency.

There is no quick route to being slim. It took a while to put it on, and it takes a while to take it off safely.

As a result of the accident that paralyzed me in my youth, my elimination organs—bladder and bowels—were less effective at moving wastes out of my body. My physician at that time told me I would have to rely on laxatives twice a week. Every Tuesday and Saturday became "laxative day" … for years. This caused two problems, at least: I was quite a bit underweight, and my effort to gain control of my muscles again was greatly delayed or slowed down. Some attempts to increase the use of my body had to be put on hold, and I was sick a lot. Seemed I couldn't even fight off a cold without ending up with pneumonia.

After several years, I found out I was aging much too rapidly. If I pressed on the pad of my thumb, it remained flat— like I remembered my grandmother's doing when she was old.

Startled, I asked the chiropractor I was seeing why this might be. She seemed a bit puzzled, momentarily, as she had no idea how I ate or that I had this laxative habit; but she gave me a book to read about nutrition, written by Adelle Davis, *Let's Eat Right To Keep Fit*. I read it from cover to cover.

Some years before this, I had read about how many calories

a body needed and had counted mine each day for a week. Well, you can imagine my surprise when I discovered I was on a slow starvation diet! I barely ate enough calories to maintain a hundred pounds—and I weighed even less than that because of the use of laxatives.

So, I picked up on my eating, but not on *what* I ate. I just ate whatever had more calories. Well, I did manage to gain weight, but as I mentioned before, I gained too rapidly. As I read the book my chiropractor had given me, I discovered that I wasn't eating enough protein to even replace the cells that regularly have to be replaced, much less build muscles. And I was not getting enough vitamin A for healthy skin and eyes—and was flushing out too much of what I did eat with my laxative habit. Oh, yes! I forgot to mention my vision had been going downhill, too, and I could scarcely see at night at all.

Between my chiropractor stimulating the nerves and muscles, and my change of diet to more fiber, water, protein, vitamins, and minerals, I was finally able to stop using laxatives. My muscle tone improved, I got colds less often, and I got over them much faster when I did.

I was thin, but I wasn't healthy. So, you can see that a study of nutrition is a *must* for a healthy body.

If you respect your body, you will give it what it requires. How long would your car run if you decided it could do just as well with sugar as with oil … or soda pop instead of water … or beer instead of gasoline? *You* won't run very well with those either. You need fresh water, complex carbohydrates and fiber from vegetables, fruits and grains, fatty acids from natural vegetable oils (one, linoleic acid, is said to be absolutely essential to life[7]), and protein, that is used to build, maintain, and repair all of the tissues of the body.

Seems like one of the first things people omit when they want to lose weight is the fats, but fat is a part of the structure of every body cell. We need fat in bile production and for the absorption of fat soluble vitamins—A, D, E, and K—and for many other functions.[8] We just need to limit it in our diet and plan our menus so we get the proper quantity of vitamins and minerals from the foods we eat.

All the above information I learned in my nutrition class at the university, as well as from Adelle Davis' book.

Let me tell you, it's mighty difficult to eat things made with sugar, that has calories but no food value, and not go over the caloric needs of the body. If you eat everything the body needs, you will find you have eaten the amount of calories needed to maintain a normal weight. If you want to eat more than that, and yet be thin, you will have to increase your activities.

In this day and age of computers, there are many good sources of information on weight and height for men and women. Rush University Medical Center has a very good table for ideal weight and height and a body mass index at www.rush.edu/rumc/page-1108048103230.html.

Look for tables that tell you how much you should weigh for your height and how many calories you burn doing different types of activities. The government has tables on line that gives the Recommended Daily Allowances (RDA) for many essential nutrients and the nutritive values of many foods. It is important that you make sure you get the proper number of calories and nutrients to sustain a healthy weight by taking into consideration your body type, activity levels, and personal lifestyle.

Some years ago, I knew a woman who was quite a bit overweight. Her regular physician happened to be out of town when she decided to go on a diet. The young doctor she queried about losing weight told her to reduce her caloric intake to less than 1,000 calories—to about 800 calories a day. I don't recall now how many days she stayed on it, but one day her daughter found her lying on a couch, unable to get up.

When her doctor got back in town, he found her in a hospital bed, having suffered a mild heart attack. After hearing about the diet, he angrily admonished the young associate. "Don't you realize her heart muscle can't get enough protein and minerals on 800 calories a day? No one should eat less than 1,000, at the very least," was overheard by my friend on the other side of the door.

Just remember, though, the amounts listed are for *healthy* people. More may be required in case of illness, lowered absorption, etc. The help of a nutritionist may be required if there are special needs.

Be sure to count the calories of *every* bite and drink that goes into your body. I recall a time in the past when I thought it wouldn't hurt anything if I ate two pieces of toast with a little oleo before going to bed. Back then, I was still eating white bread. I checked and found that each slice of white enriched bread, toasted, had 70 calories (some kinds have less). 70 X 2 = 140. Now add the oleo. One tablespoon = 100 calories. 140 + 100 = 240 extra calories a day.

Since it takes 3,500 calories to make one pound of stored fat, you can easily see it only took me about two weeks to gain a pound (240 X 15 = 3600). After about a five pound gain, I decided my toast had to go! I hadn't increased my activity level any and had been about the size I wanted to be before adding the five pounds. Good thing I stopped when I did, otherwise, I might have been 25 pounds heavier by the time a year had gone by.

Then, as now, I didn't weigh myself very often. But I knew right away I had gained about five pounds before I even stepped on the scales. How did I know so quickly that I had put on five pounds? By my clothes. A long time ago, I decided it was okay if I went down a size, but I would never buy any clothes larger than a size 12 (the size charts have changed over the years, 12 is now size 10 or less). I lived in pants, and I loved wearing jeans. Whenever the waist snap or button couldn't be fastened, I would go on a weight reduction program. A too tight pair of pants was a definite warning signal to me. I refused to put up with the discomfort for long so it always triggered weight loss before much time went by.

How many of you wear stretch waist bands, big loose dresses, or clothes designed to hide all? How many problems get solved by being hidden? Do your dishes get done while being hidden away in the oven? Do the dust bunnies under the bed finally mysteriously disappear if you drop a large enough spread over the bed to reach the floor and keep them hidden? Do the accounts total themselves while tucked away in the bottom of a desk drawer?

Get that fat out where you can see it!

Sure, there are people running around overflowing their shorts and skimpy bathing suits—but they don't want to be thin. *You* do! There's a difference. If *you* see yours, you'll be inspired to work on it. If *your* clothes feel tight, it will remind you not to eat so much. It's easy to forget about it when you're comfortable and it's well hidden. "Out of sight, out of mind." Enough said about clothes.

Yes, I could gain easily because I'm not as active as the average person. But my first husband was just the opposite. He told me he couldn't gain weight no matter what he ate, but if the calories in his diet were totaled, he would have found he ate very little more than I did at the time. "If you continue eating the number of calories needed for someone weighing 116 pounds, you'll eventually dwindle down to that—do you want to weight 116?" I asked him.

Actually, he was over six feet tall, and I'm not sure how much his bones weighed or how rapidly his metabolism worked, so it was difficult to know exactly what he'd weigh otherwise, but I think he got the picture—he started eating a little more.

Just think what would happen if you dropped two pieces of bread with oleo or butter from your daily intake, instead of adding it like I did. Remember, that was about two pounds a month. You'd hardly miss two slices of bread a day. And what would happen if you walked moderately fast for thirty minutes a day. The middle of the moderate range is about 200 calories burned per hour, so that would be 100 calories per half hour. It would add up to 3,500 calories in 35 days—just a little over a month.

See how easy it would be to lose a total of three pounds a month? That's 36 pounds a year! You just keep adjusting your activities (caloric output) and your caloric intake, until you are losing the amount you want to lose at the rate you wish to lose it. You don't have to get real physical, and you don't have to starve. It just takes being *consistent*, daily sticking-to-it, and persistence. A change of life style is what it's all about.

Remember, whenever you expend enough extra energy to burn 3,500 calories, you lose a pound. And ditto for whenever you subtract that many calories from your diet. If you eat only 120 calories less a day, it will take a month to lose one pound. But if you subtract 1,000, that's 30,000 a month—or a loss of 8 ½ pounds (30,000 divided by 3,500). But remember also, for each 10 calories eaten every day above what your body uses, you will gain one pound per year.

With the information you find on the Internet, you should be able to evaluate your present diet and make appropriate changes. As the weight comes off, you will not be hungry as often, so you need to make each calorie you ingest count towards good health. You will want to treat your body with the respect due the house of your spirit, so you can be active and healthy all the days you remain on this Earth.

And remember, action and feelings follow thought. So when you feel hunger pangs, unless it's been a *very* long time since you've eaten, it isn't *really* hunger. It's an "I want" thought. It's desire for high calorie foods: habit foods—usually junk food loaded with sugar and/or salt. And habits can be changed.

Make substitutions. Save those strongest desire-items for special occasions. Use a smaller plate ... or fill it half full, and drink that glass of water before you start. Keep a list of what you eat and drink every day for a while. Total up the calories. Total the amounts of other nutrients from the tables. Check the requirements. Then start revising what you eat. The human body was designed to work quite well as long as we give it what it needs.

In this age of people eating out at restaurants, one can usually find that most of them have basic caloric and nutritional information available at the restaurant, or on the Internet, to help them total up their intake of calories and nutrients.

Sure, I could write you out a menu—a diet. And you could follow it each and every day, and you would get what your body needs and lose weight. But you can get that kind of help anywhere.

You don't *need* more help! What you *need* is to take more responsibility for what you do. You know which foods you like best among the ones having the required nutrients. If you take the time and effort to plan a proper diet for yourself, you will see firsthand where the mistakes of the past were made and be able to evaluate proper action wherever you are.

It's kind of like riding a bicycle. As long as someone holds you up, you won't be able to get your balance and ride on your own. But as soon as that someone lets go, you may wobble for a while, but before long you're sailing along feeling great because you did it yourself!

And that's the only way to stay thin—do it yourself. You've got the will—here is the way. Read on. There are many roads leading to Thin City; besides thought and action, there is fantasy and self-hypnosis to help you attain your goal.

PART THREE

Fantasize Yourself Thin

Chapter Seven

See Yourself as You Want to Be

We get very little in this life that isn't planned for—either step-by-step planning, or in picturing it first in our minds.

When you decide to buy a new car, you shop around. You look at the cars lined up on a dealer's lot. You peer through showcase windows. You've already decided you *want* a new car; you've already checked your books to see if you have the resources to acquire one. All that remains is deciding which one you most desire—what will it look like?

Finally you see it—*your* car! It's just right for you—it's *the* one!

After you leave the showcase window in which you spotted the perfectly perfect conveyance (stores are closed—you have to wait until tomorrow to buy it), you can just see yourself behind the wheel, driving down the street, stopping at a friend's house to show off your dream buggy, and finally pulling up your driveway and parking it in your garage. Ah, yes! You can "see" the whole wonderful inner-moving-picture of it any time you close your eyes—you and your car! It's especially exciting and vivid if it's to be your first car—or, at least, the first one you plan to purchase all by yourself.

And this inner visualization of you and your car continues until you bring about the actual event of purchasing and driving your new automobile.

Whether you've ever bought a car or not, you have been a consumer of goods, so you know what it's like to purchase something new. First comes the desire to own it. Then you see the item in your mind and see yourself using it. You imagine yourself owning what you desire before you bring that event into reality. You actually cause things to happen by mentally picturing the whole process, step-by-step. By seeing each facet of the ownership in your mind, you build up desire until you just "have to have it!" then the *plan* of how to get it comes into being and is set into motion.

So, you see, you're not only a consumer; you're also an architect and a builder. An architect designs and plans—a builder carries out those plans. If the plans used by your subconscious mind to construct your body aren't to your liking, then you'll just need to revise them! You can't build a sound structure with faulty plans.

If you desire to change your body, and you visualize those changes, you can build a new you. But first, you've got to check the plans you have so you'll be aware of the changes needed.

While I attended college, working on my undergraduate degree in psychology, I met a midlife woman who was quite a bit plumper than she wanted to be. One day between classes, she told me she had discovered why she had put on all the extra weight and was now going to be able to lose it easily. "For many years now," she said, "I've been wanting to be a grandmother. I could just see myself in a big old Mother Hubbard apron, cuddling my grandchildren on my lap." During one of her self-awareness classes, she had discovered that this inner view of herself had been causing her to eat more, unconsciously, little by little, and to exercise less, so that eventually she could have this grandmotherly look she had pictured for herself. Her metabolism had slowed down. Most of the old-time pictures of grandmothers revealed them to be quite a bit heavier than today's modern grandmother wants to be—at least, the one she had picked for her model was.

Now, being aware of the problem, she had been told that in order to change her biological clock (so that the little devil with the prodding pitchfork, who sticks us in the posterior whenever we stray from our set path, will change the prodding eat-limits), she would have to change her internal image of herself. She would have to see herself in a different role ... one in which she could be thin.

She could have seen herself in the role of a model, swimming instructor, dancer, exercise leader, marathon runner, or just the foxiest-looking lady for her age anywhere—one who is pointed at when remarks like "... and she's sixty years old!" are heard.

Until she brought up the subject of our inner "clock," I'd forgotten studies in neurobiology about how our metabolisms speed up or slow down according to how our "clock" is set—and that our thoughts and view of ourselves can change it. At the time I had studied the subject, I'd been just where I wanted to be, weight wise. But by this time, I had put on a few unnecessary pounds.

So, immediately, I pictured a clock in my mind with numbers on it both below and above the weight I wanted to be, and I mentally moved the clock's hand back until it pointed to 116 pounds. Most every time I shut my eyes, I continued to check the clock and move it back if the hand wasn't pointing to 116. It didn't take long for me to lose enough weight to weigh exactly what I saw in my mind.

Of course, I've never weighed much more than my ideal weight. My view of myself has always been to be more active as I get older.

I recall a class I had on career planning. At one point in the semester, we were told to pretend we had just reached our 65th birthday and were being interviewed by the press. "And how is your life going now, Billy, and what are your future plans?"

"I've been living in Colorado Springs for some time now; I have just come in from climbing a mountain and must finish typing the manuscript for a new book the publishers are waiting for," I told the interviewer.

Several young people in the room looked at me rather oddly, as I was still hobbling around slowly with a cane, dragging one foot most of the time. Furthermore, I was already in my mid-forties and had never written a book. Some of the kids ahead of me said they were going to retire to their rocking chair in the backyard. That didn't sound like the kind of picture I wanted to put *myself* into! Sounded rather dull and self-defeating.

How can you get better if you see yourself getting worse?

And I have continuously improved each and every year since the accident that laid me low when I was eighteen. So, I don't want any of you to tell me it can't be done—or that you're already too old. No one is too old or too much out of shape to try. And that's where it all begins … with the "try." The more you try, the more you can do. There is no reason age should keep you from doing anything, if desire is a part of you.

Why, I remember reading about a man who was still climbing trees when he was well over 100 years old. I heard about another man who, through an improved diet and lots of massage and stretching, was more active and felt better in his eighties than he had in his twenties. I even heard about a nursing home in a Scandinavian country where many of the seemingly senile residents who entered the establishment were able to return to their homes after improving their diets.

Just think what *you* could do with *your* body by using a little effort, a little planning, and a little awareness of its needs— rather than your *wants*!

Ready to start visualizing a new you?

Some people tell me they can't visualize. When they close

their eyes, everything is just dark ... blank. Guess they didn't spend any time daydreaming as children. If any of you have this problem, then let's begin where you are. You need lots of practice. It wouldn't hurt those of you who *can* visualize, but for whom the pictures aren't clear and sharp, to practice a bit, too.

If you have a photo of yourself being the size you want to be, use it for your practice. If you've never been thin, then just use any picture that pleases you—or use an object such as an apple, an orange, a leaf, or a flower. Place it in front of you. Look at it intently. Study every feature. Then close your eyes for just a moment and try to "see" the object or picture. Open your eyes and look at the object again—longer this time—then close your eyes briefly and try again. Keep increasing the time spent focusing on the object. Alternate back and forth at least ten minutes the first day. If you still can't see the object clearly, try again the next day. Keep increasing the time spent each day in trying to see it as soon as you close your eyes. Work up to 30 minutes a day with your object, alternating back and forth between eyes open and eyes shut. Use the same object or picture each day until you can see it clearly in your mind when you close your eyes.

Then try another object. When you can see still-life objects clearly, try something moving. Watch a child or a dog run. Close your eyes and see the same action again. Look outside at the landscape. Close your eyes and see it. Watch someone walk by. See a rerun of the same scene in your mind. Practice makes perfect, as the saying goes. Just keep on practicing until you perfect your inner viewing.

When this has been accomplished, close your eyes and see yourself.

How do you see you? As in the photograph when you were the size you want to be ... or as you look now when you view yourself in the mirror? If you see yourself fat, then you will have to change what you "see" with your mind's eye, because when you can picture yourself thin—just the way you want to be—then those pounds will start dwindling away like magic. You will stop being hungry all the time. Your metabolism will speed up and burn calories faster. You will begin turning down food and drink that is harmful to your body and detrimental to the size you see yourself being. It all becomes so much easier once the new you is clearly in view.

Wouldn't you like that?

Okay. So create your plans—or, if you were once thin, go back to the original design. Get a good clear inner picture of yourself as a slim, healthy, active person. Picture each part of your body having this new look. Nice facial features, with prominent cheekbones; thin, well-shaped neck; you can *see* that collarbone. Lean arms; tapered fingers; you can count your ribs! Feel those hipbones! Nice flat abdomen; small hips, shapely or muscular, whichever is appropriate to your sex. Feel those kneecaps! And anklebones! See the bones in your feet! Slim and trim all over. See yourself move like you've always wanted to move. Run up the stairs and down again … in your mind. Jump. Twirl around. Isn't that great? Picture yourself doing something you've always wanted to do.

Practice seeing yourself the size you want to be, doing all the things you'd like to do, every day—many times a day.

You say you can't see yourself like that? Well, maybe you're having trouble seeing the finished product all at once. If so, start slowly and use the progressive technique.

Try this: You're in a store buying a new outfit. Picture yourself buying it just one size smaller than you wear now. Picture every detail. Choose a garment you really like to wear, hold it up to you, see the color, the texture—every detail. Maybe you've seen just what you want in a window somewhere. Pretend you're going to buy it. See yourself telling the clerk, "This is my new size. I've lost X pounds (5 or 10—however many you feel it will take for you to go down to the next size), and now this size fits great!"

Make up words you can believe, because you have to be able to believe what you tell yourself. Change the size as much or as fast as you can believe and picture ... until you can see yourself as you want to be.

Do a little daydreaming. Make up a script for yourself. You are the actor in the movie. Just be sure to see yourself slim and moving easily ... more rapidly than you do now. This is the new you.

See a clock in your mind. Set it for the weight you should be. Tell yourself, "This is my weight." See it every morning when you get up. See it again just before lunch ... and before dinner ... and before going to sleep. Every night, just before going to sleep, watch a movie of yourself doing the things you want to do, as the size you want to be. The last picture we see in our minds as we go to sleep has a much greater chance of sinking into the subconscious mind, and that's where the pattern is that needs revision. With persistence and practice, you will reach your goal. You can eventually have whatever you clearly picture each night as you drift off to sleep.

If you *do* have a picture of yourself as you want to be, place that picture where you will see it just before you go to sleep. Then study it closely each time just before you close your eyes.

Visualize yourself thin!

Right now I want you to look into your mirror and find your best physical assets. You say you don't have any? Look closer. Everyone has features that they and others find pleasing, but some people are always quicker to notice the less desirable features of their bodies. That's probably due to past criticisms. Some people get so used to being criticized, especially while growing up, that they find it much easier to accept criticism, even from themselves, than to accept a compliment.

Are *you* more used to being criticized than complimented?

And then, too, it seems there are people who just like to

focus on bad points rather than good; maybe they've watched too many news broadcasts.

If you're going to be a new you, you've got to make a few changes. One is to learn to focus on the positive. Ignore the negative. Don't be like the ostrich that sticks its head in the sand hoping whatever threatens will go away. Just shift your focus from the features you don't like to those you do. Look for the good. Do you like your eyes? Then tell yourself so. It's not being too vain or proud to like a God-given feature. If *I* gave you something, I would hope you could say, "I like this!"

So look at yourself in the mirror and say "I like my eyes," or "I like my nose," or "I like my complexion," or "I like my hair." Whichever features you like, tell yourself so.

After you pick out a number of features (assets) about yourself that you like, and have told yourself so, pay attention to other aspects. Do you like the way you *do* something, *say* things, and *write*, etc.? Pick out things you do that you like, and tell yourself you *enjoy* doing them.

Practice talking to yourself in this positive manner every day.

This practice can gradually be expanded to include other people. Look for their best features and actions. Focus on what you *like*, not what you dislike.

One problem many of you have is that you want to lose excess weight instantly. Wouldn't it be great if there were a magical potion—add water, stir, drink, and presto! Instant thinness?

But that's not the way it works. Just think about how long it took you to get to the size you are now. You can lose it faster than that, though, because you are going to work at it. You didn't work at getting fat; it just kind of sneaked up on you. But you can't lose it overnight ... or in a week ... or in a month. Even if you could, it wouldn't be safe, and you wouldn't be healthy. Embark on a continual weight correction plan that really works and will ensure you're staying at the right weight for you for the rest of your life.

Whatever you can picture yourself being is what is right for you. If you can't picture yourself as thin, then either you aren't ready to give it up (you haven't *really* made the decision), or you don't have sufficient "reason" to want to be thin. You may have to set your goal lower until then—to whatever you can visualize in your mind. Use *Fantasy*—the "F" in F.A.T.

Chapter Eight

Reprogram with Self-Hypnosis

As a final oomph to our study of how-to-be-thin, I am going to teach you how to use self-hypnosis—for two basic reasons: (1) To help you become a thin person in less time and with more ease, and (2) to learn to relax.

You'd think it would come naturally, wouldn't you? Watch members of the animal kingdom, like a dog, or a cat; they seem to know how to relax. As long as we don't pen them up, they do quite well.

For us, there's where the problems is. *We*, for the most part, are penned up!

We are enclosed by four walls, a floor, and a ceiling for most of our lives—at home, at school, or at work. We ride around in metal tubes of one kind or another. We are caught up in a race for everything, as though we were being chased—grades, jobs, promotions, deadlines, security. Get married, have a baby, buy a house, get a car, keep up with the Joneses—don't let them get anything we haven't got! Take a vacation—*hurry, hurry, hurry!* Hurry back in our tubes to our pens so we can pay for whatever fun we thought we had.

Was any of it relaxing? Did you spend much time relaxing on your vacation? Do you feel relaxed *now* ... anytime ... anywhere at all?

Yes, you'd think it would be a natural part of our lives—but it's not. We have to *learn* to relax.

As a member of a civilized society, it is necessary, at least part of the time, to be confined (or so it seems) in an enlarged cell (house, office, work place, school, conveyances), but we don't have to suffer stress because of it. We can learn to do what we feel we must in a much greater state of relaxation—and many people will find they won't eat as compulsively if they are not under pressure. But as it is, there is so much pressure it's almost, at times, as though the compulsive eaters are telling the world, "I can't control this madhouse, this situation, etc., but I can eat whatever I want to!" Of course, they aren't *really* saying it—they just reach for another this ... and another that ... and another anything.

Relaxing the body also helps all bodily functions work better. When I first learned how to totally relax all over, I discovered I had been tensing one nostril. Who knows why! Several years before, I had brought the narrowness of the one nostril to my doctor's attention. It was difficult to breathe through it; I thought it was growing together. Doc gave me a nasal spray intended to enlarge the passageway. Didn't help much, though, so I never mentioned it again—just figured nothing could be done about it. I had many worse problems at the time to worry about. My stomach hurt so badly I could scarcely eat without pain. Of course, these were actually minor complaints next to my partial paralysis, but they seemed big to me, because I had zeroed in on them. My focus was on what to do about these problems in particular, because I just didn't want any more disability than I already had.

Well, it was quite a relief—and a surprise, let me tell you—when I finally realized, while trying to relax my body completely with progressive relaxation, that I, myself, had a tight grip on these parts and was squeezing the very life out of them! If you squeeze an area tightly enough, you cut off part of its blood supply, and it slowly loses function or dies. All tissues of your body have to be fed in order to live.

Why would I do this? Who knows? The "why" didn't matter as much to me as the fact that I was doing it. Knowing that, I could stop. When I learned to relax those areas, I could breathe easier and eat without pain. I didn't have to find out "why" in order to change the behavior.

Over the years, I learned a great deal about how we tense first this part of the body and then that part—unconsciously. Why, we can shut down part of the veins or restrict the nerves leading to our hearts, ears, eyes, throat, breasts, hands, feet—any part of us—and cause them to react oddly or have difficulties. We could make our hearts beat more rapidly, become hard of hearing, prevent our breasts from enlarging as we grow, have cold hands and feet, or we could create an endless array of other problems without ever being aware that we caused them ourselves. Why, we can even prevent a doctor's medicine from doing us any good, if we do not desire to get well.

A psychology professor I studied under during my university years told of an episode that happened to him in his youth that clearly demonstrated the power of our minds over our bodies.

I won't go into the details of his physical problem, but he had to undergo a number of very painful operations. He spent a lot of time in the hospital and had been given many shots of morphine for the excruciating pain. Being a very bright young lad, he spoke to his dad one day about his fears of becoming addicted to the morphine, since he would still require so many more shots in the future.

His dad immediately voiced his concern to the doctor in charge. "No need to worry," said the physician, "we aren't really using morphine; it's just a placebo. There is absolutely no way he could become addicted."

Straightaway Dad hurried to inform his young son that he

had nothing to worry about; they were not using morphine on him—it wasn't anything at all, actually. Well, dear old Dad really messed it up for the kid that time! Now that the youngster knew it wasn't really a "pain shot"—that had worked beautifully up until then—it no longer worked. From that day forward, the young lad felt the terrible pain of it all because they had nothing strong enough to knock it out, except morphine, which they didn't dare use over such a protracted period of time.

Yes, the mind has power over the body. Sometime, somehow, we put the message into our "computer-brain"—our subconscious mind—to tense parts of our body, for whatever reason. *You* are tensing parts of your body, too. And you can stop it! That's where self-hypnosis comes in.

Why hypnosis instead of just relaxation exercises alone? It is because you relax more completely during hypnosis, and you can reprogram your "computer" at the same time.

Hypnosis is a sleep like condition very near the sleep level of consciousness. One is still aware of surroundings at this level but does not pay attention to them. And one is more receptive to suggestions; hence, the openness to reprogramming.

Why *self*-hypnosis instead of just going to a hypnotist? When you pay someone else to help you, you have to go back … pay again … and again ... and again. It usually takes a series of sessions to be of adequate help. And then you won't know how to use it later without going back for more help, because you've given the control to someone else. Each of us needs to learn *self-control*. I'd rather suggest things to myself—follow my own counsel—than listen to the suggestions of another when I'm in a receptive state of being.

Those who learn to hypnotize themselves can use the technique on various occasions throughout their lives. It can be used to break habits, control pain, correct physical problems as well as for relaxation and weight control. Once you learn to relax your body, you can go to sleep faster and require less sleep, because you rest so much better. And you can get more fully in touch with your own mind and its abilities. We don't really use much of the mind's power. What is it they say—we only use about ten percent of our ability, more or less?

So, let's just start right in. The sooner we start, the sooner you'll become aware of what you have been doing to your body while you weren't paying attention. And you'll begin shedding those unwanted pounds with ease.

First, select a quiet place. Turn off your phone. Make sure the clock won't suddenly chime or cuckoo next to you. In other words, you don't want to be disturbed for at least fifteen minutes once a day. Later, the time may be increased.

In order to get the feeling of being relaxed, I want you to practice progressive relaxation. We will begin with the toes. Tense the toes of both feet. Curl those toes under tightly; tense your feet as much as you can. Hold it for a count of five. Now relax them. Utterly relax all your toes and both feet. *Feel* the difference. Doesn't it feel great to relax them?

Now tense both legs. Harder! Hold the tension at least five counts, and then relax both legs all at once—completely. Tense both hips. Hold for five. Relax and *feel* the difference. That's what we're after here—the difference. You need to know how each part of your body feels when it is relaxed.

Tense your abdomen ... as tight as you can. Hold. Relax. Tense your chest ... and back ... and stomach. Hold. Relax. Wonderful to relax, isn't it?

Tense your hands. Make two fists ... very tight! Hold. Relax. Tense both arms. Draw them up to your shoulders. Hold. Relax and let them drop to your lap or side. Next, tense your shoulders. Shrug. Scrunch down your head and neck into your shoulders as though you were trying to hide them between the humps. Hold for the five, and then relax. Really drop them all of a sudden. Let go! Ah, sooo relaxed.

Now tense your neck, throat, lower jaw. Clinch your teeth.

Hard! Hold. Relax. Drop your lower jaw—separate them until there is a little space between your teeth. Lots of people find that the main areas they often tense, unconsciously, are the shoulders and the jaws.

While studying biofeedback, I met a young man who had been working with the equipment for some time. He told me to especially check for tension in the jaws. He had discovered that tension there was the cause of headaches he had been having.

"As soon as I see the prices on items in the grocery store," he said, "I have to immediately drop my lower jaw and open my mouth. If I don't, I get a headache before I leave there. Sometimes I get rather strange looks from the clerks and other customers; they don't often see such clear demonstration of awe at the rapidly rising prices."

The other customers were probably afraid to look at the prices after seeing his reaction. During times of inflation, many people clench their teeth and tightly clamp their jaws together as they shop. Any time you find you have done so, open your mouth as wide as you can and then relax it leaving the teeth slightly apart.

Now, squeeze your eyes tightly shut. Scrunch up your face. Purse your lips. Squeeze your nostrils together. Hold. Relax. Be sure to relax the muscles around the eyes.

Frown. Tense your forehead. Hold. Relax. Tense your scalp. Hold. Relax.

Work on tensing and relaxing, alternately, for fifteen minutes. That's what I want you to do the first day. Just become aware of which parts of your body you tense regularly and how they feel when they are relaxed, so that when you want to relax you will immediately know the feeling to assume.

Second day (or second period of the same day), again make sure you won't be disturbed. It would be best if you sit in a straight chair—one in which your spine will be straight. Some people recline while hypnotizing themselves, but more people than not tend to go to sleep when they lie down and relax. If you put a baby into its bed to play, then later expect it to go right to sleep when you lay it down, you may find it doesn't want to go to sleep.

Conversely, if you get used to going to sleep when you try to hypnotize yourself, you'll not be able to do it in any position. And it only takes a few times of drifting off while trying to go down into a hypnotic sleep to make a pattern and establish a habit of regular sleep instead of hypnosis. Remember, hypnosis is very close to the sleep state.

Okay. So ... you're sitting in your chair. Put your feet flat on the floor—never cross your legs or your feet. Put your hands palms down on your thighs—never on the arms of the chair. During hypnosis, the body relaxes so much you could cut off circulation to areas in uncomfortable positions. Some people turn their hands palms up, but I find palms down to be more natural. Try it both ways. Do you feel a pull in your shoulder or arms with palms up? When you stand up, which feels more comfortable, palms back or palms facing forward? My body feels best with palms back when standing with arms down at my sides ... which would be same as down on my thighs.

All comfortable now?

Slow your thoughts down. How? Well, just refrain from thinking about anything; focus on your feelings instead of thinking of external things. Thoughts may come in, but withdraw your attention from them and focus on your body.

Close your eyes (naturally, you will have read and reread this part until you have the sequence memorized before you begin). Take several very slow, very deep breaths. Breathe so that your abdomen moves in and out. Abdominal breathing (expanding the diaphragm and abdomen with each inhalation) is much more relaxing than when sucking in the diaphragm and expanding the chest as you inhale. In fact, any time you feel yourself becoming upset or tense, for whatever reason, take several deep abdominal breaths. Really expand and contract that abdomen in a nice, slow, regular rhythm. This calms you down faster than anything else.

Focus on the rhythm of your breathing awhile. Now turn your attention to your feet. If you have practiced your progressive relaxation sufficiently, you will know how to relax them and how they feel when relaxed. Say to yourself, "I am relaxing my feet." Follow that in a couple of seconds with, "They *are* relaxed." Then focus on the calves of both legs. Repeat the sentence, but insert "calves" in place of feet. "I am relaxing my calves; they *are* relaxed." Continue up the body.

"I am relaxing my thighs ... they *are* relaxed." Then hips ... abdomen ... lower back ... stomach ... chest ... upper back ... arms ... hands ... shoulders. Remember, when you get to the shoulders—or any other part of your body that you tense more often than other parts—to say, after the usual "I am relaxing my shoulders ... they *are* relaxed," that they are "feeling very loose" or "they are *very* relaxed." Give them a little extra time; talk to them a bit more if they need it.

My neck is relaxing ... my throat is relaxing; they are relaxed. My jaws are relaxing; they are relaxed. My nostrils are relaxing ... they are relaxed. My eyes are relaxing; the muscles around my eyes are relaxing ... they *are* relaxed. My ears are relaxing ... they are relaxed. My forehead is relaxing; it *is* relaxed. My entire scalp is relaxing; it *is* relaxed.

"I am relaxed all over."

Practice this progressive exercise each day in the same place, preferably about the same time of day, until you can relax easily, quickly. Then try skipping the first half of each statement—the "My feet are relaxing." Try going straight to "My feet *are* relaxed," etc., right on up the body. Actually, by the time you've learned how to relax each part as you focus on it, exclusively, it then becomes just a process of checking to see that all of you *is* relaxed—that you're not tensing one part or another.

Whenever you feel enough time has been spent on relaxing muscles—when you can do it well and rapidly—then I want you to go through the steps of closing your eyes, breathing in rhythm, and relaxing the body. After you tell yourself "I am relaxed all over," then I want you to begin at the top of your head and pretend you are draining the last little bits of tension down through the body and flushing it all out. Silently tell yourself, "Any remaining tension anywhere in my head is going down ... down into my neck." *Feel* it go down. Picture a fluid going down, if that is easier. The main thing is to get the feeling of going "down." Also, it will actually "drain" out any tension you may have missed. Later, you will go rapidly through this stage, too, as a final check and to get in touch with a "going down" feeling.

Take the fluid, or just the draining-down feeling, through the neck, into the shoulders, down through the arms, down to the hands, and drain that tension (or fluid) out through the fingertips. Tell yourself you are draining the tension "down ... down through the chest ... down through the stomach ... down through the back ... down through the abdomen ... down through the hips ... down through the thighs ... down through the legs ... down through the feet ... and on out through the toes." Be sure you feel it flowing down through each part as you name it, and be sure to say "down."

"My body is completely drained of all tension. I am totally relaxed."

Some people may already be able to do this. Others may take a few days, a week, or several weeks. Practice until you can accomplish a feeling of utter relaxation easily—and the feeling of "down."

Now you're ready to really go "down" into a hypnotic state and get in touch with your subconscious mind. Some people worry that they may become hypnotized and not be able to come out of it. Nothing to fear. You would just sleep for a while and wake up as though from a nap.

Okay? Ready? There are many ways to go into trance. Here's one: You've just drained all the tension out. Picture yourself in your own backyard or in the park. There is a swing. Sit in it and begin to swing. Big, high, back-and-forth swoops! Begin swinging as fast and as high as you choose. After a little while, begin slowing down. Slower ... slower ... slower ... until you can bring the swing to a complete stop.

Here's what that does: it slows down your brain's rhythm. You begin fast in beta, slow to alpha, and then to low alpha or theta brain waves. I have been connected to an electroencephalograph (EEG—a device used to discern and record the electrical activity of the brain) while doing this exercise and have reached a hypnotic "dream" state by the time the swing was stopped. The slower the brain's rhythm, the closer you are to sleep—delta waves. Theta is the state just before you drift off to sleep—a kind of half-sleep. One may see visions or dream while not actually asleep, yet. The idea is to hold that state of consciousness without going on to sleep.

One way to do that is to make sure you're not in your usual sleep position (which is usually lying down) and to focus on something as soon as the proper state is reached.

To hold that state of consciousness, talk to yourself or imagine images of your choice as soon as the swing stops. You shift your attention from the swing to whatever you wish to program into your "computer"—or reprogram. It's like that last thought or picture before going to sleep. Your mind works to bring about what you feed into it just before you go to sleep. The mind doesn't sleep. Might as well accomplish something you want to accomplish instead of just weaving dreams off and on all night. Of course, you'll still dream, but you might have some clearer, more distinctive, learning dreams—answers could come to you during the night—or during your hypnotic session. Some people drift a little deeper after their self-programming and have a creative or learning dream that helps them with their lives and increases their creativity.

Back to the programming, our main concern now is to be thin and healthy. So when you reach the deepest stage of hypnosis you can reach, without going so deep you will forget to talk to yourself, start giving yourself suggestions. These should be made up beforehand, written down, and memorized. Make up your own program to feed your computer-mind.

For example, you might tell yourself the following: I eat 1200 calories (or however many you decide) a day—no more, no less; I feel satisfied and comfortable eating only 1200 calories a day; I eat *only* natural, health-producing foods that are good for my body; I drink eight glasses of water every day; I drink *only* health-producing drinks, like water, milk, and juices; I am becoming more active; I walk 20 minutes each day after my main meal; I sleep no more than eight hours each night.

Just make a short list and silently tell yourself as many as you wish, or can remember, each time you reach the proper level of relaxed state. Repeat the same ones each day.

Immediately after making the "I" statements, picture yourself the size you want to be, doing things you will be doing as soon as you have reached your goal. Picture yourself getting on the scales; see yourself at your target weight (or a lower-than-now weight). *Feel* the excitement of reaching your goal. See yourself dressed as you'd like to be. Tell someone in your inner movie about how excited and happy you are to be the size you see yourself.

In order to program your mind to bring about the desired results, you have to feed it pictures of what you want—the finalized product—with appropriate words and feelings.

All of this should not take over fifteen minutes; however, you may want later to increase the time to thirty minutes. After the program has been inserted, you can either bring yourself back to full alertness or go a little deeper and perhaps dream a dream of helpfulness.

If you wish to go deeper, silently tell yourself, "I am now going to go down deeper and dream a short dream that will be of help to me in understanding my life and situation." If there is a specific situation you wish help with, mention it to yourself. Then say, "With each count, I am going down deeper—deeper, deeper, down—and will dream a short dream. In five minutes, I will come back up to this level after the dream." Then begin to count *slowly* backwards from five to one after telling yourself you will begin dreaming on the count of one.

Dreaming may not be reached the first day, but if you continue to repeat the same thing every day right after programming, you will eventually begin having helpful dreams.

When you come back up to the pre-dream level—or if you chose not to go deeper after programming—it is time to come back to full alertness. Tell yourself, "When I count from one to five I will be alert, awake, and feeling great. One—two—three—four—five. Up! Awake! Feeling great!"

It doesn't matter whether you count forwards or backwards at each step, or whether you count three, five, or ten each time. Whichever you feel comfortable doing, that's how many and in which direction you should count. The mind works on what you suggest to it. However, I always count backwards because you are less apt to hear backwards counting while out about doing everyday activities such as driving.

Each time these steps are repeated, you will feel so much better. So relaxed. So refreshed. And it won't be long before you will begin to notice a big difference in your life … and size.

After coming back up, take a few minutes to reorient yourself before getting up out of your chair. When you get to the point where you stay down thirty minutes or more, your heart will have slowed down quite a bit. You need to stretch and come fully "awake" *slowly* before arising (you may even want to take 5 or 10 minutes). It's kind of like getting up in the morning, except you will feel lots better than you usually feel then.

Your mind should be instantly alert as soon as you think the last "Feeling great!" with emotion, but your body will awaken a little more slowly. If any part of you remains somewhat numb, as though it were still asleep, either wait a bit or *tell* it to wake up.

I recall one time I was practicing my self-hypnosis when my husband wanted my attention outside where he was building steps at the back of the house. He didn't know I was "down." Since in trance you may hear things going on around you and yet are not really paying attention to it, I heard his call but ignored it because I wanted to stay down. His call had partly aroused me, though, as when someone calls you when you are asleep. You may partially wake up, but, being terribly sleepy, you want them to go away so you refuse to come fully awake. If they stop calling, you may not even remember that they called.

But then I heard him tell our oldest son to go in and get me to come outside. Hearing this brought me to the realization that I was going to have to get up, but I felt real sluggish, like being awakened in the middle of the night. So I quickly went back to the feeling of being "down" and told myself, "When I count from one to five, I will be awake, alert, and feeling great. One— two—three—four—five. Awake! Feeling great!" and, presto! I felt *great!*

Then, too, here's another method for going "down": After you relax completely and drain, see yourself going down steps. Count them as you go down. Tell yourself there are ten steps, and you are going to be in a hypnotic sleep when you get to the bottom—step number one. *See* yourself going down the steps. .*Feel* yourself going down the steps while you count ten—nine— eight—seven—six—five—four—three—two—one.   Count *slowly.* When you get to one, immediately begin your programming. Each time you practice, you will go a little deeper.

Another method is to see yourself in a lovely, relaxing environment. Some prefer a sandy beach. If you do, see yourself lying in the sun on the sand with the warmth of the sun relaxing you. Tell yourself you are sinking slightly into the sand. Say to yourself, "I am warm. I'm so relaxed I'm sinking into the sand. I'm *so* relaxed." Repeat it quietly several times. Just continue to *feel* the heat of the sun as you lie there, until you feel there is nothing in the world but this delightful, relaxed, warm feeling. Then begin programming.

Some see themselves sitting under a favorite tree—lying on the grass—in a haystack. Wherever you feel comfortable and at peace (and can see yourself relaxing there) can bring about the hypnotic state.

Some people are so easily hypnotized that they can just tell themselves they will be in a deep hypnotic state at the count of three, and can then give suggestions to the subconscious mind.

Others can stare at themselves in a mirror until their eyes feel heavy and tired. By telling themselves they will be in a deep hypnotic sleep as soon as they close their eyes, it is accomplished. And others stare at a candle's flame ... or the fire in a fireplace.

You might even practice just focusing on your deep rhythmic breathing, and tell yourself you will go deeper with each exhalation of breath.

The main thing is to find a way to stop thinking about all the things one normally thinks about. "Stop your thoughts. Make your mind a blank. See a blank screen in your mind," was the advice I was first given. Of course, when you can get the blank screen, you can write your own ticket—draw your own pictures, or just wait to see what will be drawn upon the screen for you by your inner self. But it took me a lot of practice using the first two methods described here before I could get to the blank screen.

Some of you may not be sure when you've reached the proper level of "down" before programming. One way I tell is when I've lost awareness of my body, or when I can't tell whether the fingers of my hands were touching each other or not before I started.

Many people have the wrong idea about hypnosis. Of course, a hypnotist can take you to a deep level from which you may not remember anything you heard unless the hypnotist tells you to remember it. But you are also in a light trance state when you watch one thing so long you lose awareness of the rest of the world. Some people are hypnotized by the dividing line on a highway while on a long trip; others react similarly to a windshield wiper blade and may even have an accident because their attention has been withdrawn from their driving.

Kids are often hypnotized by the TV—grownups, too. You can be hypnotized by watching something like sand falling through an hourglass, the movement of a metronome, the steady sound of the ocean surf, raindrops beating against the roof or windowpane, or by some types of music.

Haven't you ever stared at something so long you weren't aware of things going on around you or listened to music until you were in a reverie of your own?

Many children don't hear Mother call while they are daydreaming. A light hypnotic trance (which is all that's needed for programming) is just the withdrawal of the attention—the perception—from the world around you and focusing on the world *within* you … the inner visions. Here's where it all begins … and then extends outward where others can see what you've been inserting into *your* computer.

Yes, self-hypnosis can be a valuable tool. Just like everything else a person wants to do well, "Practice makes perfect."

Well, maybe none of us are perfect and most likely never will be during our stint here on Earth, but we can, with a little concerted effort each and every day, become better caretakers of our bodies than we are now.

Did I hear someone out there say, "I don't have time for all that!'"?

Do you have time to be ill? Do you have time to spend sitting in doctors' offices, or lying in a hospital bed? How much time does living right really take? Fifteen minutes of relaxation—maybe thirty. Let's say thirty. One week totaling calories and nutrients to see what changes need to be made. With calorie charts and a calculator, it only takes about fifteen to thirty minutes at the end of the day to improve your life. So far, we've got about an hour, then a twenty minute walk twice a day—that's forty minutes. Changing thought patterns—thinking—you do that anyway, so that doesn't take extra time. Moving faster should eventually give you *more* time, because it will take a lot *less* time to do whatever you do all day ... but, we won't subtract anything for that because you may decide to walk wherever it is you go each day instead of riding in a car or on a bus. And again, you should be needing less sleep by the time you've practiced relaxation, visualization, and hypnosis.

You may spend thirty minutes visualizing, too, so if we don't subtract anything at all that comes to just a little over two hours a day. Isn't your life worth that? Isn't your body?

Why, if all you do to improve your body only increased your life by ten years, that's 87,600 more hours to live. The two hours you spend each day to accomplish that only adds up to 730 hours a year. Why, you'd have to live 120 more years to spend *that* many hours working at having a healthy, more active life! And what do you accomplish with the time you *think* you save by *not* doing these things?

Just think of all the benefits! Less illness. Less money spent on doctors, hospitals, and medicine. Those are just some of the savings. The best part is how you'll *feel*. You'll be lighter on your feet—and no more swollen ones. You'll have more energy, sleep sounder and awaken more refreshed—even with less sleep. You'll be more relaxed and peaceful, and just think about your self-image for a moment!

How can you love yourself if you don't deem yourself

worthy of love? Obviously, you don't think you are worthy, or you would—right? If you loved yourself, you would take good care of yourself, wouldn't you? You *do* take care of others you love, don't you? Well, we're not playing "Twenty Questions" here; nevertheless, it's essential to make a point. In order to feel worthy, you have to do something for which you can be proud of yourself. A job well done. Finishing something you start. Accomplishing something important that everyone feels is quite difficult to do.

What better way to increase your worth—your self-image—than by accomplishing what you *really* want ... to be thin! You *do* want to, or you wouldn't have read this book. If you've been for a ride on the *Merry-Go-Round* (diet syndrome), your self-image has taken a real beating. How could it not?

It's about time to reverse the trend, isn't it?

Someone else wrote your program, pressed your buttons, and now you're like a robot. You buy what TV says to buy. You fix it according to the directions on the package. Some of you think you're watching your weight by drinking diet-pop instead of the sugared kind—if you disregard the chemicals and dyes, they don't hurt anything ... or do they? But you drink it—just because someone told you to on TV.

Aren't you tired of being ordered around by a set you bought in the first place? Or by the ads paid for with the money you've spent all these years buying junk food? Wouldn't your self-esteem really soar if you took charge and told them all to go to ... and stay put?

Aren't you willing to put forth a little effort ... starting right now?

Your efforts toward changing your lifestyle by using F.A.T. will be richly rewarded ... by the slim, healthy person who flirtatiously winks back at you as you pirouette in front of your full-length bedroom mirror one day in the not-too-distant future.

PART FOUR

How to Raise Thin Kids

Chapter Nine

Child Abuse

How dare sadistic creeps sexually molest the children of this world! How *dare* overgrown bullies maliciously beat the little ones!

We let out a scream of protest that's heard around the world when anyone dares to harm one of our kids—or anyone else's.

Yet, there is someone abusing most of them every single day of their lives!

Child abuse is not only that which is done *to* them but also that which is *not* done. Brutality can break bones; sexual molestation can affect the mind; neglect can do both.

Some will protest loudly, "What do you mean, neglect! Why, I give my child *everything*!"

Giving too much is sometimes part of the problem, but what concerns me most is what you may *neglect* to provide, do, or teach. Have you neglected to teach good eating and drinking habits, teach basic concepts of health, teach self-responsibility, teach patience, teach coping techniques, teach them how to relax, and set a good example? Have you or anyone else bribed your child instead of doing any of the above? If so, then you're guilty of child abuse.

If *you* don't teach these things, who will? And if no one does, your child will suffer from this neglect all through life.

Raising a child entails more than just giving birth and providing food, shelter, and security.

Do you put on rose-colored glasses when you look at your child so you won't see any flaws that may be just beginning to surface because of such neglect? As the saying goes, "There are none so blind as those who refuse to see."

Open your eyes! Take off those glasses and take a good look. Parenthood is not a profession to be taken up lightly. It requires thought, study, knowledge, work, dedication, persistence, patience, and, most of all, love. It takes planning, supervision, and constant watchfulness. It must not be a hit-or-miss affair—your child's *life* is at stake! That little body is being formed from the ingredients you provide. It's your responsibility to help your child set the foundation for a structure that will last in good condition, hopefully, for a hundred years. And not only must the building be sound in its structure, but also the child must be taught how to maintain its soundness and strength after the building of it is completed.

For a moment, pretend you are a building inspector. Look at your child as critically (but don't criticize) as you would an apartment building that is being erected with your money and in which you are going to live.

Look at the overall outward appearance—the surface. Is the skin clear of blemishes, eyes bright, vision sharp, hearing good, hair shiny and manageable, nails strong, and teeth free of cavities? Check the substructure. Bones of the legs straight? Back straight? Digestion good? Heart normal? Check the ventilation. Breathing deep and regular? Check the wiring. Is the child calm—not over-active or nervous? Check general functioning. Is the child alert? Active? Does the child sleep well at night? What about habits? Is there a disciplinary problem? How about coping ability? Can the child handle stress and frustration? Any known health problems?

If your evaluation has unearthed a problem, or if you are

planning to have a baby, I strongly recommend that you do research into the nutritional needs of children. You can't end up with a brick building if you build it with straw.

If your child is overweight but still in fairly good shape health wise, check the RDA requirements for your child's age and height and make a thorough evaluation of the diet you are providing. Is the child consuming excess calories beyond present needs, either in food or drink? Be aware, too, of food intake at baby-sitters or day care/nursery school. Plan the days' menus so that the child obtains the proper number of calories, proteins, vitamins, and minerals according to age and height. Overeating sometimes results from the lack of a required nutrient.

School age children should be allowed to help plan the day's food intake. Let them go over the charts with you. Discuss dietary needs with them—and which foods they can choose from—so they will know how to eat right when you're not there. They need to know *why* they must eat food that provides plenty of calcium and protein and what happens to their bodies when they don't eat properly. The more they learn about how their bodies work, and which nutrients are essential, the more likely it is that they will eat properly for the rest of their lives ... and the healthier they will be for it.

One of the greatest gifts you can give your child is the gift of knowledge—the "how to" and the "why" of it all. You can help children become health conscious, but you don't mold a child. You guide and provide for basic needs. A child is like gelatin. You provide the bowl, add water (proper nutrients), pour the mixture into the mold, set it in the refrigerator (proper environment); but it's time and the inherent nature of gelatin that brings about the final shape. If the right amount of water is added, it will hold its shape once the bowl (parents) has been removed. If the mixture is weak from over dilution (overindulgence), then it will fall apart and be a shapeless mass or even turn to jelly when support is withdrawn.

Yes, gelatin has the potential to be pretty resilient stuff, but it can easily be weakened if one doesn't know how to work with it. You do the child no favor by giving in to every demand. A child isn't just born with the knowledge of what the body does or does not need. If children could be born self-sufficient, what would they need *you* for? It took you quite a while to learn what you know, and you're still learning, so why expect the child to know how to choose a proper diet for optimum health? Leave out just one ingredient and a health problem will eventually be the result.

For example, when I was in my thirties, my husband and I decided to adopt twins—a boy and a girl. They were nearly seven years old when we took them out of the orphanage, and they both had nutritional deficiencies. Vicki had frequent nosebleeds with the least provocation. She could be sitting quietly in the back seat of the car on the way to church, to visit Grandma, or to shop and suddenly spring a gusher all down the front of her dress. After many trips home with pinched nostrils to change clothes and put ice on the back of her neck, we found she was deficient in vitamin C (found in citrus fruits), bioflavonoids (found in the white around the orange), and chlorophyll (found in dark green leafy vegetables like spinach).

Besides that, I was handed a bottle of liquid medicine as I left the orphanage with instructions on how much and how often to give it to Vicki for asthma. She had just recently been in the hospital for a rather severe attack.

But when my doctor checked her over, he very wisely told me not to mention to her that she had asthma, or it might become a crutch or a "big stick" to be used to get attention or her own way. He also said that the medicine wouldn't prevent an attack. All she knew, at the time, was that she had been sick.

So I put the medicine on a shelf and waited to see what would develop. I didn't want her to get into the habit of taking medicine unless it was absolutely necessary; I'd heard at that time, that asthma was usually more emotionally than physically induced.

Before long, Vicki had an attack in the middle of the night. It is frightening to watch a child struggle to breathe and see the difficulty of it bring a look of fear to her eyes. For a moment, I wondered if I should give her the medicine—but if I did, I knew she would make the connection between breathing difficulties and taking medicine, and from then on she might become a cripple, so to speak.

I knew that what she *really* needed was to learn how to relax and breathe properly so that a hospital-requiring future dependency wouldn't develop.

So I spent the rest of that night in a chair beside her bed. First, I placed one hand on her abdomen and held one of her hands with my other. Then I told her to breathe with me in a regular, slow rhythm—deep, slow, abdominal breaths—in and out, making sure her breathing moved my hand sufficiently. I kept telling her to watch me breathe and to breathe with me. I smiled to show her I wasn't frightened, and I kept telling her, "It's okay—relax and breathe with me."

Naturally, if she had gotten worse instead of better, I'd have been on the phone to Doc, but as I slowed my breathing down, so did she, and before long she was fast asleep. I stayed upstairs with her that night just so I could reassure her if she woke up.

It was the first and last asthma attack Vicki ever had after coming to live with us, and the medicine was tossed out at the end of that first summer.

But, the little boy's problems took a bit longer to overcome. Rick was terribly thin, weak, and uncoordinated, and he was hyperactive and just couldn't sit still. Some part of his anatomy was on the move constantly!

As I left the orphanage with him, I was told by the mental health professional who checked him over that it was an emotional problem. He gave me the name of a tranquilizer I should have my doctor prescribe for Rick, and he told me to tell his teacher not to try to make him sit still—it would be impossible.

Again, my doctor said the tranquilizer would not *cure* the problem and would create a dependency. He advised against it, and I concurred.

Furthermore, I did not speak to his teacher about his problem because that would have set him apart from the other kids as being "different." I didn't know what kind of future problems that might create, and I felt certain I would find a way to solve his hyperactivity before long, anyway. My doctor had advised me to monitor his diet to see if there might be nutritional deficiencies.

Much had been learned by watching animals, and there were lots of them around to watch. We had a mink farm back in those days, and we had learned a lot about nutritional needs of our animals. It seemed to me then (and still does) that more attention was given to the diets of both farm animals and pets than to the diets of those caring for them and their families. Our animals had to have a vitamin and mineral supplement such as vitamin A for healthy skin and glossy hair, and B-complex and magnesium for calm nerves—mink become overexcited easily. And we included wheat germ oil during breeding season to "up" the kit (baby mink) average per female and to produce healthy young from eager-to-breed adults.

Besides the mink at the time, we had an old blond Cocker Spaniel dog that had been hit by a car some years before. He had suffered some neurological difficulties and had stopped his frequent visits to the female dogs in the neighborhood. We didn't know whether he *couldn't* perform the sex act or just wasn't inclined to anymore. But the first spring after we began adding the wheat germ oil to the mink food (that was his daily diet, too), he began chasing again and was never without his females from that year until his death.

We had also learned to add brewer's yeast, which is an excellent source of B vitamins, to the pregnant females' diet, and we had the calmest, best nursing mink mothers of any ranch in the Midwest.

Since magnesium had also been found to be necessary for nervous animals, I decided to see what it would do for Rick. With Vicki having been deficient in several nutrients, I was pretty sure Rick's diet could stand some improvement too. Along with an improved diet, the effect of 500 mg. of magnesium a day, with his doctor's approval, was dramatic. Rick calmed right down. And between that and the Canadian Air Force exercise program we put him on, his coordination improved from kicking himself on the insides of each leg as he ran, with head and arms flopping hither and yon, to a darn good gymnastic athlete in high school. He went from the little boy who fell exhausted at my feet, nearly unable to catch his breath after just one trip around the house, to a Rugby player by the time he was grown.

Of course, 500 mg. of magnesium was double the RDA for Rick's age. But he had been deficient for a long time, and it took a while to correct both the problems caused by that deficiency and to change his eating habits—at that time, the magnesium was discontinued. Too much magnesium can cause diarrhea.

Yes, a dietary deficiency of any of the numerous nutrients required by our bodies will eventually cause illness and weakness. Sometimes the effects become noticeable in a very short period of time.

When my husband was a very young child, small bald spots began to appear, periodically, on first one part of his scalp and then another. He would lose all the hair from a space about the size of a nickel—sometimes larger. Variable amounts of time would pass, and eventually the bald spots would fill back in with new hair growth. By the time he reached school age, the shiny bald spots became embarrassing to him, as they might appear in front, on a side, or on the back of his head. Hair was worn very short in those days, and the spots were quite noticeable as often as not. Melvin grew up during the Great Depression of the thirties, and his family was often in need of food and clothing— no one in his environment had money to spend to solve the riddle-of-the-bald-spots. So he just silently suffered the humiliation and worried that he might someday lose even large chunks of hair.

By the time we married, he had gotten fairly used to the affliction. Feeling that there must be something a doctor could do, I urged him to see a specialist. He did. But, besides relieving him of a pocketful of money, the doctor and the treatment prescribed did not do one iota of good, as far as the spots were concerned.

The doctor had given Melvin extremely large doses of vitamin A for several months, as he felt positive there was a deficiency.

Well, he was right about the deficiency of A, but the treatment was incomplete. Quite a number of years later, I learned from reading the Adelle Davis book that vitamin E must be taken with vitamin A, and both are oil soluble and have to be taken with a meal containing fat.[9] So, once again he tried vitamin A, but this time he took it along with vitamin E at mealtime. And, according to Adelle Davis, the treatment of a deficiency of vitamin A could take as long as four months or more before results would be noticeable, so sometimes failing to get the desired results may be caused by ceasing treatment too soon.[10]

Guess what! He never had another bald spot the last fifteen years of his life. If he had been a lover of carrots and wheat germ, or even fresh whole wheat, he never would have had the problem. He may have been too poor to get what he needed in his youth all of the time, but ignorance of dietary needs kept the condition going until midlife.

Some people considered Adelle Davis somewhat radical. However, by reading her books I became more aware of nutritional deficiencies and requirements and began to pay more attention to my own diet and that of my children. It is best always to use caution and check with a licensed nutritionist.

Yes, our children must be taught as much as possible about good nutrition while they are still in our care in order to prevent health problems now, as well as later in life. Deficiencies are preventable with a little forethought and planning.

But many kids get several times what they need ... and *don't need*! If yours is in this category, the next chapter is for you.

Chapter Ten

The Overindulged Generation

Look around you! Look at all the overweight kids! Does anyone care that these kids are suffering ... and *will* suffer from all the overindulgences?

Everywhere I go, kids are being handed candy. In banks. In stores. From Santa Claus to *Trick-or-Treat*, and in between, it's considered good business to indulge the children of present and potential customers. The person who said, "The way to a man's heart is through his stomach," should have included, "... and the stomachs of his children."

One old saying is being taken quite seriously: "Love me, love my children." Boy! Is that one ever being taken advantage of—from the politicians who kiss the babies to the trip to Disney Land my daughter won at a local grocery store. Store owners know kids will beg for candy while Mom waits in line if it's placed at cart height near the checkout stand.

And everyone knows a little kid will stop crying if you hand out a sucker. But why not a balloon? Store owners' names and advertisements would be given wide exposure when stamped on a free balloon and carried down the street by small hands. And think how much better that would be for the little ones' health and teeth. Caring moms would appreciate it more, too. But, as it is, if children play their cards right, they can collect enough bribes and sweet tidbits from everywhere Mom goes to either become addicted to sugar with the possible health problems or become grossly overweight by the time they start to school ... or both.

What's to be done? Do you care?

If so, then join me in the most unpopular exercise of the vocal cords. Practice saying "No!" the word "no" is one letter less than "yes" and very easy to say ... with practice.

Of course, they'll scream. But it'll be good for both of you. The kids will learn some appetite control, and you'll learn patience and assertiveness. When you say "yes" when you know the answer should be "no," you lose your position as one-who-guides, which is the position all parents should fill. You become a "yes-man," a follower rather than a leader, not the guardian and guider of youth you should be.

The best time to start is today—right now. Habits are formed very early in life, so you can't start too soon.

Make some rules about what your child may eat at home and elsewhere. Tell the child what the rules are. Tell the grandparents, aunts, uncles and friends. Of course, it's best to begin when the child is very small so good habits will be established before the child starts to school, but, whatever the age, start *now*!

Some rules you might establish are as follows: Dessert is reserved for special occasions such as Christmas, Easter, birthday, or maybe Sunday dinners—but only then after the main courses; food may not be taken from strangers (that includes people downtown, even when Mom's along); food will not be eaten between meals (and that includes while riding in cars). Soda, artificially sweetened drinks, and candy are all empty calories that are not necessary (and some have dangerous ingredients)—fruit juices, fruit and natural foods will be substituted.

Kids who are used to eating raisins and nuts prefer them to candy, and will continue to unless their parents allow candy and artificially sweetened drinks as the children gain more exposure to society.

Yes, the word "no" is a necessary part of your vocabulary if you want thin, healthy kids. It gets easier the more you say it. Each time you use it, though, once said is sufficient. Then practice ignoring the pleas—no matter how loudly expressed. Over time, the protests will cease. After all, it took a while for them to become demanding and it will take a while to undo the damage.

As you get used to enforcing the eating rules, try branching out into other areas of child guidance. Pay attention to how much TV your kids watch. Actually, that's where they learn some of their unhealthy eating habits.

I recall the first summer after adopting the twins. They could name all seven ways certain bread builds strong bodies— or whatever the commercial was. They could recite it word for word. Too bad they didn't know one for whole wheat bread instead of white, because it took me awhile to get them turned around on that one. They kept begging me to buy the brand in the commercial, but white bread, to me, looks anemic and tastes like cardboard (probably stems from my knowledge of what it lacks nutritionally).

Besides being brainwashed diet-wise by the TV, too much time spent in a sedentary position slows the metabolism so that it takes less food to get fat. And the imagination isn't exercised as it is when a book is read. You picture the action in your mind as you read instead of having it all done for you.

Too much TV also cuts down on physical activity that burns calories and strengthens bodies. So, make rules about TV viewing. Limit it to so much time per day and let the kids choose between appropriate programs .The same should apply to the computer after homework is done. That helps teach self-control and responsibility. Making choices needs to be learned early in life. Always give children choices to make in order to strengthen their coping skills. They need to learn early in life that there are choices to be made and they have to make some of them.

If children get everything they want early in life, they will either decide the world owes them what they want, and take it if it isn't given, or become morose and despondent when they can't get it later on ... or even become suicidal. You won't always be with them to take care of all the wants, so don't make your children any more dependent upon you than is necessary.

And besides, half the fun in life is the expectation, the excitement, the looking forward to something. If one is given everything early in life, what is there left to look forward to? Where is the incentive to be on one's own and work towards a goal?

So, don't give them everything and take away the delicious anticipation and satisfaction of doing it for themselves. Don't feed them so much they lose pride in *self*. Don't bribe them with food or anything else—that's the easy way out. Don't compare them to anyone else; each child is unique in its own way. Comparison creates resentment—and resentment creates all kinds of problems including poor eating habits.

Be a good example in everything you do by exerting self-control. Children are great imitators. Don't be a tempter or temptress; if food or drink is not nutritious it should not be in your house. Fat parents most often raise fat children due to their own lack of good dietary choices. And if you're not active, it's less likely your children will be active.

Do promote the drinking of water. All too often children live through an entire day with a little milk here, a little juice there, and lots of soda or other sweet drinks in between. Where's the water? Water is a basic need for children as well as adults and very often greatly neglected.

Do watch your language when you speak to, or about, your

children—you are describing them for them (ref: Part One).

Treat them as you would treat your friends … and they will be friendly. Treat them with tenderness, affection, and love, and they will be loving and caring—most welcome additions to a peaceful society and the Universe.

ABOUT THE AUTHOR

Billy Branson had an auto accident in 1950 that resulted in paralysis from the neck down due to a spinal cord injury. She had been married only 9 months, and was 18 years old. She went on to awaken her body and walk again.

Billy was married to her first husband for 50 years before his death and is currently married for the second time. During her life, Billy has raised 3 children, earned a B.S. in psychology, an M.S. in counseling and has become an ordained Spiritualist minister. She was certified in clinical hypnosis and conducts workshops to train hypnotherapists. Billy has studied astrology for many years. These skills were combined and used in her private counseling practice.

Having worked with many overweight women, Billy is quite qualified to help others become thin, be thin and stay thin for the rest of their lives!

Other books by Billy Branson:

Mining The Silver Lining, Taking Triumph from Tragedy

How Astrology Saved My Life, Learn My Simplified Method to Gain Health, Wealth and Understanding

Works Cited Endnotes

[1] Ask A Biologist. Building Blocks of Life, Shyamala Lyer, "Cell Division." September 27, 2009. ASU School of Life Sciences. August 1, 2013 <http://askabiologist.asu.edu/content/cells-divide>

[2, 3] William Shakespeare, *Hamlet*, Nunnery Scene, "Hamlet's Soliloquy - To be, or not to be." Act 3, Scene 1, line 56.

[4] Doctor Oz. < http://www.doctoroz.com/videos/sleep-type-your-personalized-plan-fight-disease> March 11, 2013, "Study from the Perelman School of Medicine at the University of Pennsylvania." Dr. Michael Grandner, "Calcium Loss at Night." February 6, 2013.

[5] International Journal of General Medicine. doc 10.2147/UGM.S 18837. Yasuyo Hijikata and Seika Yamada, "Walking just after a meal seems to be more effective for weight loss than waiting for one hour to walk after a meal." June 9, 2011 <http://www.ncbi.nlm.nih.gov/pmc/articles/PMC3119587/>

[6] The USGS Water Science School. Howard Perlman, "The Water in You." August 9, 2013. USGS. January 4, 2014 <http://ga.water.usgs.gov/edu/propertyyou.html>

[7, 8, 9, 10] Davis, Adelle. *Let's Eat Right to Keep Fit*. New York City: Signet Books, 1970.